# *In vitro*
# Experimental
# Pharmacology

# In vitro
# Experimental Pharmacology

**Asmita Gajbhiye Patil** M Pharm, PhD
Professor
Department of Pharmaceutical Sciences
Dr Harisingh Gour Vishwavidyalaya, Sagar, MP

**Shailendra Patil** M Pharm, PhD
Professor and Dean
Faculty of Pharmacy and Medical Sciences
Swami Vivekanand University, Sagar, MP

**Shweta Mishra** MS Pharm
Research Scholar
Department of Pharmaceutical Sciences
Dr Harisingh Gour Vishwavidyalaya, Sagar, MP

**Debashree Das** M Pharm
Department of Pharmaceutical Sciences
Dr Harisingh Gour Vishwavidyalaya, Sagar, MP

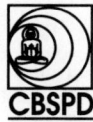

CBSPD

## CBS Publishers & Distributors Pvt Ltd

New Delhi • Bengaluru • Chennai • Kochi • Kolkata • Lucknow • Mumbai
Hyderabad • Jharkhand • Nagpur • Patna • Pune • Uttarakhand

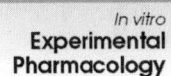

*In vitro*
**Experimental Pharmacology**

**ISBN:** 978-93-88178-93-8

Copyright © Authors and Publisher

**First Edition:** 2019
**Reprint:** 2024

**CBS Publishers & Distributors** Pvt Ltd
4819/XI Prahlad Street, 24 Ansari Road, Daryaganj, New Delhi 110 002, India.
Ph: 23289259, 23266861          Website: www.cbspd.com
                                e-mail: delhi@cbspd.com
*Corporate Office:* 204 FIE, Industrial Area, Patparganj, Delhi 110 092
Ph: 4934 4934        Fax: 4934 4935    e-mail: publishing@cbspd.com; publicity@cbspd.com

*Branches*

- **Bengaluru:** Seema House 2975, 17th Cross, K.R. Road,
  Banasankari 2nd Stage, Bengaluru 560 070, Karnataka
  Ph: +91-80-26771678/79          Fax: +91-80-26771680          e-mail: bangalore@cbspd.com
- **Chennai:** 7, Subbaraya Street, Shenoy Nagar, Chennai 600 030, Tamil Nadu
  Ph: +91-44-26680620, 26681266          Fax: +91-44-42032115          e-mail: chennai@cbspd.com
- **Kochi:** 42/1325, 1326, Power House Road, Opp KSEB, Ernakulam 682 018,
  Kochi, Kerala, India
  Ph: +91-484-4059061-65          Fax: +91-484-4059065          e-mail: kochi@cbspd.com
- **Kolkata:** 147, Hind Ceramics Compound, 1st Floor, Nilgunj Road, Belghoria,
  Kolkata 700 056, West Bengal, India
  Ph: +91-33-25633055/56          e-mail: kolkata@cbspd.com
- **Lucknow:** Basement, Khushnuma Complex, 7-Meerabai Marg
  (Behind Jawahar Bhawan), Lucknow 226 001, UP, India
  Ph: +0552-4000032          e-mail:tiwari.lucknowi@cbspd.com
- **Mumbai:** PWD Shed. Gala no. 25/26, Ramchandra Bhatt Marg, Next to JJ Hospital
  Gate no. 2, Opp. Union Bank of India, Noorbaug, Mumbai 400 009, Maharashtra, India
  Ph: 022-66661880/89          e-mail: mumbai@cbspd.com

*Representatives*

- **Hyderabad** 0-9885175004 • **Jharkhand** 0-9811541605 • **Nagpur** 0-8692091830
- **Patna** 0-9334159340 • **Pune** 0-9664372571 • **Uttarakhand** 0-9716462459

*Printed at* Glorious Printers, Daryaganj, Delhi, India

*to* _____

*whatever the mind can conceive*

*it can achieve*

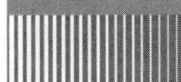

# Preface

**B**ehind even the most stunning success stories lie countless unsuccessful attempts. Even in case of drug discovery science, almost every day a fellow researcher conceptualizes some or the other form of medication that would be viable against the deadliest form of maladies plaguing mankind, however, only a mere handful finds its way to the commercial setting. One of the most important hindrances in translating a laboratory created medicine into successful clinical practice is lack of the comprehension of its pharmacological profile. *In vivo* animal experimentations require exquisite variety of skill and more importantly a strong ethical jurisdiction justifying the use of a fellow living being is such trying setting as that inflicted during the course of animal studies. The first edition of 'Laboratory Manual of *in vitro* Experimental Pharmacology' is an integrated compilation of concise background information and directions for activities, including experimental protocols to be performed in pharmacological laboratories that would not necessitate the use of an actual animal. The protocols described would enable a researcher to again an insight into the possible biological activity possessed by the test compound. The assays illustrated in the book are simplistic in approach and would be an effective prelude justifying whether or not to instigate further *in vivo* studies. The book describes procedures that are easy to understand and can actually be performed in laboratory setting without the use of animal model. The experiments explain the basic principles therein, e.g. effects of the test on target proteins, enzymes and cells, thereby aiding students in understanding drug target interaction.

**Asmita Gajbhiye Patil**
**Shailendra Patil**
**Shweta Mishra**
**Debashree Das**

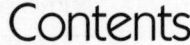

# Contents

*Preface*                                                                 *vii*

*Colour Plates*                                    *Between pages 84 and 85*

**1. Introduction to Experimental Pharmacology**                           **1**

**2. *In vitro* Anti-inflammatory Assay**                                 **14**

    2.1  To study the *in vitro* anti-inflammatory potential of the given sample against heat-induced protein denaturation *17*

    2.2  To study the *in vitro* anti-inflammatory potential of the given sample by membrane stabilization assay (heat-induced hemolysis) *19*

    2.3  To study the *in vitro* anti-inflammatory potential of the given sample by membrane stabilization assay (hypotonicity-induced hemolysis) *21*

    2.4  To study the *in vitro* 5-lipoxygenase inhibitory potential of the given sample using 5-lipoxygenase inhibition assay *23*

    2.5  To study the *in vitro* hyaluronidase inhibitory potential of the given sample using hyaluronidase inhibition assay *25*

    2.6  To study the *in vitro* anti-inflammatory potential of the given sample by COX inhibition using luminescent assay protocol *29*

    2.7  To study the *in vitro* COX inhibition potential of the given sample by using oxygen uptake assay protocol *32*

    2.8  To study the *in vitro* COX inhibition potential of the given sample by using peroxidase assay *35*

    2.9  To study the *in vitro* COX inhibition potential of the given sample by using prostaglandin E2 enzyme-linked immunosorbent assay (PGE2 ELISA) *37*

**3. *In vitro* Antioxidant Assay**                                       **41**

    3.1  To study the *in vitro* antioxidant potential of the given sample by DPPH scavenging activity *42*

    3.2  To study the *in vitro* anti-inflammatory potential of the given sample by hydrogen peroxide scavenging ($H_2O_2$) assay *44*

3.3 To study the *in vitro* antioxidant potential of the given sample by nitric oxide scavenging activity *46*

3.4 To study the *in vitro* antioxidant potential of the given sample by reducing power method *48*

3.5 To study the *in vitro* antioxidant potential of the given sample by total antioxidant capacity assay (phosphomolybdenum method) *50*

3.6 To study the *in vitro* antioxidant potential of the given sample by ferric reducing antioxidant power (FRAP) assay *52*

3.7 To study the *in vitro* antioxidant potential of the given sample by xanthine oxidase activity *54*

3.8 To study the *in vitro* antioxidant potential of the given sample by hydroxyl (HO˙) radical scavenging assay *56*

3.9 To study the *in vitro* antioxidant potential of the given sample by superoxide radical scavenging assay *58*

**4. *In vitro* Antidiabetic Assay**                                             **60**

4.1 To study the *in vitro* antidiabetic potential of the given sample by determining its α-amylase inhibitory action using starch iodine method *63*

4.2 To study the *in vitro* antidiabetic potential of the given sample by α-glucosidase inhibitory assay *65*

4.3 To study the *in vitro* antidiabetic potential of the given sample by glucose diffusion assay *67*

4.4 To study the *in vitro* antidiabetic potential of the given sample by protein tyrosine phosphatase inhibition assay *69*

4.5 To study the *in vitro* antidiabetic potential of the given sample by glycation inhibition assay *71*

**5. *In vitro* Enzyme-Based Assay**                                             **74**

5.1 To study the *in vitro* protease inhibitory potential of the given sample using protease inhibition assay *75*

5.2 To study the *in vitro* tyrosinase inhibitory potential of the given sample using tyrosinase inhibition assay *78*

5.3 To study the *in vitro* acetylcholinesterases (AChE) inhibitory potential of the given sample using acetylcholinesterases inhibition assay *80*

**6. *In vitro* Antimicrobial Assay**                                             **82**

6.1 To study the antimicrobial sensitivity of the given sample using Kirby-Bauer method *94*

6.2 To study the antimicrobial sensitivity of the given
    sample using Stokes method *100*

6.3 To determine the minimum inhibitory concentration
    (MIC) of the given sample using broth dilution method *103*

6.4 To determine the minimum inhibitory concentration
    (MIC) of the given sample using agar dilution method *106*

6.5 To determine the minimum bactericidal concentration
    (MBC) of the given sample using broth dilution test *108*

6.6 To study the *in vitro* β-lactamase inhibitory potential
    of the given sample using β-lactamase inhibition assay *110*

**7. *In vitro* Assay for Tropical Disease**                          **112**

7.1 To study the *in vitro* antimalarial activity of the given
    sample by using 72 hours *in vitro* growth inhibition assay *131*

7.2 To study the *in vitro* antimalarial activity of the given
    sample by using hemozoin-based colorimetric method *133*

7.3 To study the *in vitro* antimalarial activity of the given
    sample by using candle jar method *136*

7.4 To study the *in vitro* activity of the given sample
    against leishmaniasis using leishmanicidal assay *138*

**8. *In vitro* Anticancer Assay**                                    **140**

8.1 To study the *in vitro* antimitotic potential of the given
    sample using *Allium cepa* root tip assay *143*

8.2 To study the *in vitro* antimitotic potential of the the given
    sample using germination assay *146*

8.3 To study the *in vitro* MTS cytotoxicity assays *150*

8.4 To study the *in vitro* MTT cytotoxicity assays *152*

8.5 To study the *in vitro* apoptosis by estimation of DNA
    fragmentation *154*

8.6 To study annexin A5-induced apoptosis
    (annexin A5 affinity assay) by flow cytometery *159*

8.7 To study annexin A5-induced apoptosis
    (annexin A5 affinity assay) by confocal
    scanning-laser microscopy (CSLM) *163*

8.8 To study *in vitro* apoptosis by TUNEL assay *166*

8.9 To study the antiangiogenic activity of the given
    sample by chorioallantoic membrane assay (CAM) *177*

8.10 To study the antiangiogenic activity of the given
     sample by endothelial cell tube formation assay *180*

*Index*                                                              *187*

# CHAPTER 1

# Introduction to Experimental Pharmacology

The term 'pharmacology' as we understand it today seems to have been defined for the first time in 1791 by a German chemist and physician Friedrich Albrecht Karl Gren (1760–1798) when he distinguished between 'pharmacology as the science of the action of drugs' and 'materia medica as the description and collection of drugs'. Pharmacology can be defined as the study of the effects of drugs on the function of living systems. The origin of pharmacological research can be traced back to the second half of the 19th century when their founders Rudolf Buchheim and Oswald Schmiedeberg investigated the action of existing drugs in animal experiments. With the emergence of synthetic chemistry the pharmacological evaluation of these products for therapeutic indications became necessary. The classical way of pharmacological screening involves sequential testing of new chemical entities or extracts from biological material in isolated organs followed by tests in whole animals, mostly rats and mice but also higher animals if indicated. Most drugs in use nowadays in therapy have been found and evaluated with these methods. Also, developments in the area of *in vitro* techniques have substantially transformed the facet of drug discovery. While it previously took weeks or even months to test a sample for some assays, it can now take only a few hours.

## BIOASSAY

Bioassay or biological standardization is defined as estimation of the concentration or potency of a substance by measuring its biological response in living systems. The relative strength of the sample under study is determined by comparing its effect on a test organism with that of a standard preparation. Bioassay or biological standardization is a type of scientific experiment typically conducted to measure the effects of a substance on a living organism and is essential in the development of new drugs and in monitoring environmental pollutants. Both are procedures by which the potency or the nature of a substance is estimated by studying its effects on living matter. Bioassay is a procedure for the determination of the concentration of a particular constitution of a mixture.

Bioassays are procedures that can determine the concentration of purity or biological activity of a substance such as vitamin, hormone, and plant growth factor. While measuring the effect on an organism, tissue cells, enzymes or the receptor is preparing to be compared to a standard preparation. Bioassays can be classified in two types:

- Qualitative
- Quantitative

**Qualitative bioassay** is used for assessing the physical effects of a substance that may not be quantified, such as abnormal development or deformity. Example of a qualitative bioassay includes Arnold Adolph Berthold's famous experiment on castrated chickens. This analysis found that by removing the testes of a chicken, it would not develop into a rooster because the endocrine signals necessary for this process were not available.

**Quantitative bioassays** involve estimation of concentration/potency of a substance by measurement of the biological response it produces. These bioassays are typically analyzed using the methods of biostatistics.

## Principles of Bioassay

- Bioassay involves the comparison of the main pharmacological response of the unknown preparation with that of the standard.
- The reference standard and test sample should have same pharmacological effect and mode of action, so that their DRC curve run parallel and their potency ratio can be calculated.
- The test solution and standard should be compared for their established pharmacological effect using a specified pharmacological technique.
- The method selected should be reliable, sensitive, and reproducible and should minimize errors due to biological variation and methodology. (Animals should of same species, sex and weight and number of animals should be large enough to permit statistical analysis.)

## Need of Bioassay

1. Bioassays not only help to determine the concentration but also the potency of the sample. Potency denotes activity of the compound, i.e. if a

compound shows better activity at minute concentration, greater is the potency, and if its activity is low at lower concentrations, lesser is the potency.

2. It is used to standardize drugs, vaccines, toxins/poisons, disinfectants, antiseptics, etc. as these are all used over biological system in some form.

3. These also help determine the specificity of a compound to be used. For example, penicillin is effective against gram-positive but not on gram-negative. Testing of infected patient's sputum helps determine which antibiotic should be preferably prescribed for quick recovery.

4. Certain complex compounds like vitamin B-12 which can't be analyzed by simple assay techniques can be effectively estimated by bioassays.

5. Sometimes the chemical composition of samples is different but has same biological activity.

6. For samples where no other methods of assays are available.

*Types of Bioassays*

Basically there are two types of bioassays as per the technique used in determination of the sample under test.

1. Graded response assay
2. End-point or quantal assay

## Graded Response Assay

In this type of bioassay on increasing the dose of the drug, equivalent rise in its response is observed. The potency is estimated by comparing the test sample responses with the standard response curve. The graded dose

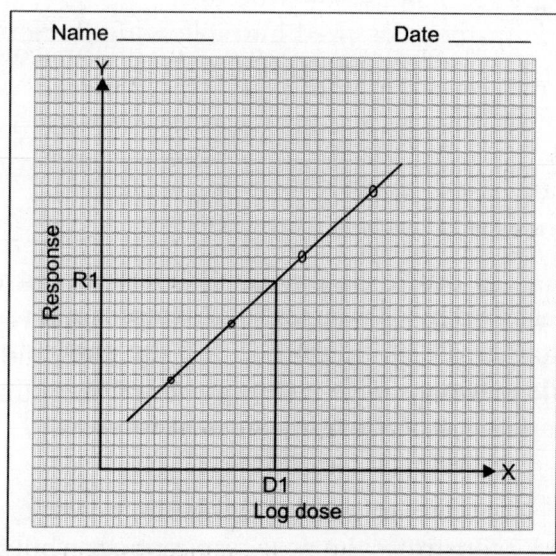

**Fig. 1.1:** Curve representing dose–response relationship

response relationship, relates the size of the response to the drug in a single biologic unit. As the dose administered is increased the pharmacological response also increases and eventually reaches a steady level called the ceiling effect, beyond which there will be no further increase in response even with an increase in dose.

The graded dose response curve is obtained by plotting a graph with dose on the X-axis and response on the Y-axis. It is usually sigmoid in shape however the log dose response (LDR) curve is almost a straight line and particularly useful in bioassay.

Conc. of unknown = Threshold dose of standard/Threshold dose of test
× Conc. of standard

Concentration of unknown is read from a standard plot of a log dose response curve of at least four submaximal concentrations.

### End-point or Quantal Assay

It is the simplest type of the bioassay. The threshold dose of the sample required eliciting a complete or a particular pharmacological effect is determined and compared with standard. For example, evaluation of cardiac effect of digitalis. Here the sample effect is identified by the response it produces on the biological system. Digitalis produces cardiac stimulation on further doses it produces cardiac arrest. Another popular example is muscle relaxant effect of (+) d-tubocurarine (TC) in rabbit.

Even the determination of LD50 (LD, lethal dose) or ED50 (ED, effective dose) is done by graded point assay procedure. Based on the method used, graded bioassay is further classified into following three methods:

1. Matching point or bracketing method
2. Interpolation assay
3. Multi-point bioassay
   - Three-point (2 + 1) assay
   - Four-point (2 + 2) assay

1. **Matching point or bracketing method:** Here a constant dose of the standard is bracketed by varying dose of sample until an exact matching between the standard dose responses and the particular dose response of the sample is achieved. This technique is used:
   - When concentration of the test sample is too less.
   - Margin of error difficult-to-estimate.

   **For example:** Histamine on guinea pig ileum, posterior pituitary on rat uterus. Figure 1.2 illustrates the dose response curve plotted in matching point or bracketing method.

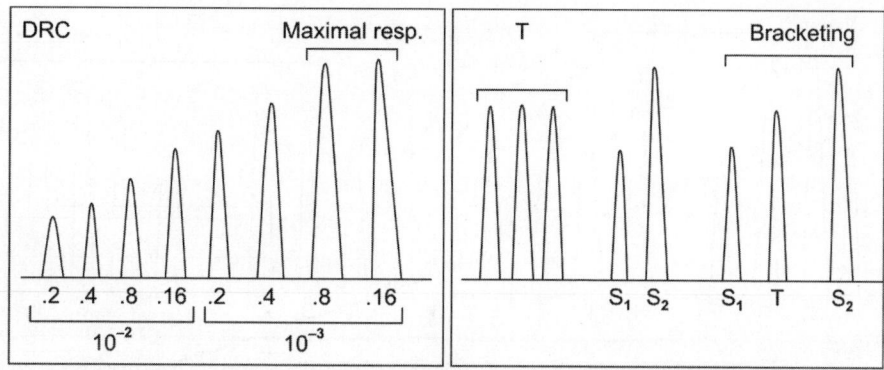

**Fig. 1.2:** Dose–response curve (DRC) for matching point or bracketing method

2. **Interpolation assay:** Bioassays are conducted by determining the amount of preparation of unknown potency required to produce a definite effect on suitable test animals/organs/tissue under standard conditions. This effect is compared with that of a standard. The concentration of the test is then obtained from a log dose–response curve plotted of a standard.

3. **Multi-point bioassay:** This method incorporates the principle of interpolation and bracketing. 2 + 1 indicates—two responses of standard and one response of test respectively. This procedure of 2 + 1 or 2 + 2 is repeated 3 or 4 times based on the method with crossingover of all the samples. It can further divided as 3-point, 4-point and 6-point bioassay.

   • *Three-point assay [2 + 1 dose assay]* is fast and convenient:
      – Log dose response curve plotted with varying concentration of standard drug solutions and given test solution
      – Select two standard doses $s_1$ and $s_2$ (in 2 : 3 dose ratio) from linear part of LDR (let the corresponding response be $S_1, S_2$)
      – Choose a test dose $t$ with a response $T$ between $S_1$ and $S_2$
      – Record 4 sets data as follows:

| $s_1$ | $s_2$ | $t$ |
|-------|-------|-----|
| $t$ | $s_1$ | $s_2$ |
| $s_2$ | $t$ | $s_1$ |
| $s_1$ | $s_2$ | $t$ |

*Log potency ratio (M) = $[(T-S_1)/(S_2-S_1)] \times log$ (dose ratio)*

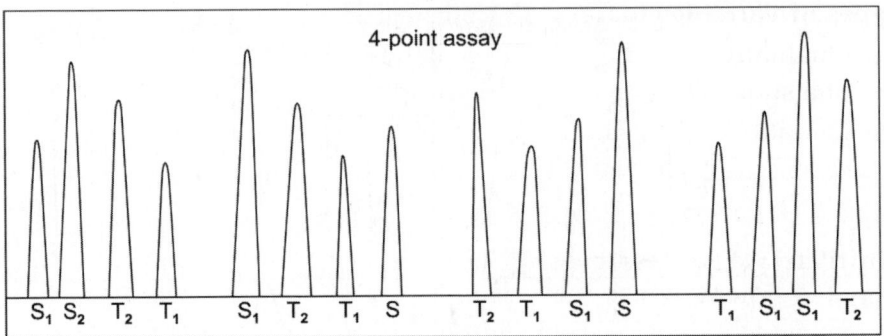

**Fig. 1.3:** Dose–response curve for 4-point bioassay method

- *Four-point assay (2 + 2 dose assay)* [For example: Acetylcholine (ACh) bioassay]
  - LDR curve plotted with varying concentration of standard ACh solutions and given test solution
  - Select two standard doses $s_1$ and $s_2$ from linear part of DRC (let the corresponding response be $S_1$, $S_2$)
  - Choose two test doses $t_1$ and $t_2$ with response $T_1$ and $T_2$ between $S_1$ and $S_2$, such that:

$$s_2/s_1 = t_2/t_1 = 2/3$$

  - Record 4 data sets as:

| | | | |
|---|---|---|---|
| $s_1$ | $s_2$ | $t_1$ | $t_2$ |
| $s_2$ | $t_1$ | $t_2$ | $s_1$ |
| $t_1$ | $t_2$ | $s_1$ | $s_2$ |
| $t_2$ | $s_1$ | $s_2$ | $t_s$ |

Figure 1.3 illustrates the dose–response curve for 4-point bioassay.

## STATISTICS IN PHARMACOLOGY

Pharmacology routinely employs statistics to help summarize data and, more importantly to test hypotheses.

**Data and variables:** 'Data' is a collective term for information gathered under various headings or variables. Variables may be related to demographic characteristics, disease specific parameters, such as the presence of coronary disease, or severity of breathlessness; or treatment response variables, such as reduction in pain and improvement of disease.

- **Types of variables (data) collected**
    i. Qualitative (or categorical) data; these characterize a certain quality of a subject (e.g. gender, age group, or disease severity group).
    ii. Quantitative (or continuous or numerical) data; these represent a specific measure or count (e.g. heart size, blood pressure, or heart rate).

- **Multivariate regression techniques:** Tools to explore relationships among following set of variables:
    i. *Dependent variables:* Response variable predicted by independent variables.
    ii. *Independent variables:* Predictor or explanatory variables which separate the independent contribution of response variables.

- **Measures of central tendency**
    i. *Mean:* The mean can be calculated by summing all the values of observations and dividing by the total number of observations.
    ii. *Median:* The median is the value that divides the distribution into equal numbers of observations.
    iii. *Mode:* The mode is the value that occurs most frequently.

- **The normal distribution:** In medical research, most quantitative variables have a range of values that occur with the highest frequency at a mean value and less frequently further away from this mean value, yielding a symmetric, bell-shaped frequency distribution. This is known as a normal distribution.

**Statistical interference:** Statistical inference is the measure of properties of the sample (such as the mean and standard deviation) and use these values to infer the properties of intervention. Based on the assumption of no bias or confounding in an ideal clinical trial, statistical inference assesses whether an observed treatment difference is real or due to chance. Strategies that are often used to make statistical inference are:

i. Hypothesis testing
ii. Confidence intervals (CIs)

- The purpose of significance or hypothesis testing is to assess the evidence for a difference in some outcome between the two groups, while the CI provides a range of values around the estimated treatment effect within which the unknown population parameter is expected to be with a given level of confidence.

- Both P-values and CIs for the main outcomes should be reported in an analysis report. Any statistical inferential results are subject to two types of errors: Type I (false positive) and type II (false negative).

**Comparison of survival data:** In clinical research, an end-point is often the time to the occurrence of some particular event, such as the death of a patient. These types of data are known as time-to-event data or survival data. However, the event of interest need not be death, but could be some other well-defined event, such as the first episode of malaria in a vaccine trial or the end of a period spent in remission from a disease. The outcome could also be a positive event, such as relief from symptoms. Survival analysis is the study of the duration of time to the occurrence of event outcomes, and is a means of determining the influence of covariates on the occurrence and timing of events. It is a set of techniques that utilizes all of the information on survival time, including censored (or incomplete) data.

**Nonparametric and parametric analysis:** Survival analysis is the study of the duration of time to the occurrence of event outcomes, and is a means of determining the influence of covariates on the occurrence and timing of events. It requires analysis of two functions of central interest, namely:
- *Survival function, $S(t)$,* is the probability that the survival time of an individual is greater than or equal to time $t$.
- *Hazard function, $h(t)$,* represents the instantaneous event rate at time $t$ for an individual surviving to time $t$.

Two methods are available to estimate the survival function:
- *The parametric method:* A particular survival distribution is assumed.
- *The nonparametric method:* It does not require any presumption of a survival distribution.

**Nonparametric analysis:** In actual applications, the population survival distribution is rarely known and hence nonparametric approach to describe the data, as it does not require any presumption of a survival distribution. Methods of nonparametric approaches involve the Kaplan-Meier method and Log-rank test.

## The Kaplan-Meier Method
- Most common nonparametric method.
- Estimates the proportion of individuals surviving at any given time in the study. When there is no censoring in the survival data, the KM estimator, $S(t)$ is the probability that an event time is greater than $t$.

Therefore, when no censoring occurs, the KM estimator, $S(t)$ is the proportion of observations in the sample with event times greater than $t$.

- **Procedure:** Rank the event times in ascending order.

Determine the number of individuals at risk and the number of events at each time. At each time $t_j$, there are $n_j$ individuals who are said to be at risk of an event and $d_j$ be the number of individuals who have an event at time $t_j$.

The KM estimator is calculated using the following formula:

$$S(t_j) = [(1-d_1)/n_1] \times [(1-d_2)/n_2] \times \cdots \times [(1-d_j)/n_j]$$

where, $t_1 \le t_j \le t_k$.

## *Limitations of the Kaplan-Meier Method*

- As survival rates are calculated throughout the study, a decreasing number of subjects will be available for follow-up as the curve progresses with time. Therefore, near the end of the study, when we have a relatively small number of subjects who have survived and are still at risk, the data are less representative of the overall effect and some sensible cut-off is needed in order to represent the data.
- The KM method is a descriptive statistical approach and therefore does not estimate the treatment effect. To establish whether there is any significant statistical difference in the survival rates between the treatment groups, a statistical test is required.

## Log-rank Test

- The main purpose of this test is to calculate the number of events expected in each treatment group, and to compare this expected number of events with the observed number of events in each treatment group if the null hypothesis is true.
- **Procedure:** Pool the two groups and sort the event times in ascending order.

Determine the number of individuals at risk and the number of events at each time in each group, as well as in the two groups combined. At each time $t_j$ $(t_1 \le t_j \le t_r)$, we assume there are $n_{1j}$, $n_{2j}$, and $n_j$ individuals at risk of the event and $d_{1j}$, $d_{2j}$, and $d_j$ individuals who have had an event in groups 1, 2, and the two groups combined, respectively.

Calculate the expected number of events and the variance of $v_{1j}$ at each time $t_j$. The expected number of events is given by:

$$e_{1j} = n_{1j} - d_1/n$$

Calculate the log-rank statistic using the following formula:

$$U_L = \Sigma \, (d_{1j} - e_{1j})$$
$$V_L = \Sigma \, (v_{1j})$$
$$\chi^2 = U^2_L / V_L$$

where $\chi^2$ is a chi-squared statistic that follows chi-squared distribution with one degree of freedom.

This $\chi^2$ value is converted to a P-value.

*Limitations to the Log-rank Test*

- It does not provide a direct estimate of the magnitude of treatment effect.
- It is mainly used to compare groups on the basis of a single variable, such as treatment.
- It is more likely to detect a difference between groups when the risk of an event is consistently higher for one group than another, but it is unlikely to detect the difference when survival curves cross.

## SCIENTIFIC CITATION

A citation is a reference to a published or unpublished source. It is important to properly and appropriately cite references in scientific research papers in order to acknowledge your sources and give credit where credit is due. Science moves forward only by building upon the work of others. There are, however, other reasons for citing references in scientific research papers. Citations to appropriate sources show that you've done your homework and are aware of the background and context into which your work fits, and they help lend validity to your arguments. Reference citations also provide avenues for interested readers to follow up on aspects of your work, they help weave the web of science.

**Definition:** Scientific citation provides detailed reference in a scientific publication, typically a paper or book, to previous published communications which have a bearing on the subject of the new publication.

**Aim:** The purpose of citations in original work is to allow readers of the paper to refer to cited work to assist them in judging the new work, source background information vital for future development, and acknowledge the contributions of earlier workers.

**Significance:** Academic writing requires the author to support their arguments with reference to other published work or experimental results/ findings. A reference system will perform three essential tasks:

- Enable you to acknowledge other authors' ideas (avoid plagiarism).

- Enable a reader to quickly locate the source of the material you refer to so they can consult it if they wish.
- Indicate to the reader the scope and depth of your research.

## Contents of Citation

Citation content can vary depending on the type of source and may include:
- *Book:* Author(s), book title, publisher, date of publication, and page number(s) if appropriate.
- *Journal:* Author(s), article title, journal title, date of publication, and page number(s).
- *Website:* Author(s), article and publication title where appropriate, as well as a URL, and a date when the site was accessed.

### Style of Citation

Referencing styles are established systems of referencing with consistent rules. Style of referencing is classified as parenthetical and numbered styles.

In parenthetical, or author-date styles, in-text references are given within parentheses before the full stop of the sentence containing the reference. APA, Harvard, and MLA are parenthetical reference styles. In numbered styles, sources are referred to with Arabic numbers within square brackets or in superscript, and the references are listed in a numbered reference list after the text. References are numbered in the order in which they first appear in the text. Vancouver is an example of numbered style of referencing.

- *Harvard style of referencing:* Harvard is a generic term for any style which contains author-date references in the text of the document, such as (Smith 1999). There will also be a list of references at the end of the document, arranged by authors' names and year of publication. There is no official manual of the Harvard style; it is just a generic term for the many styles which follow that format.
- *American Psychological Association style (APA):* APA style originated in 1929, when a group of psychologists, anthropologists, and business managers convened and sought to establish a simple set of procedures, or style rules, that would codify the many components of scientific writing to increase the ease of reading comprehension. As with other editorial styles, APA style consists of rules or guidelines that a publisher observes to ensure clear and consistent presentation of written material. It concerns uniform use of such elements as selection of headings, tone, and length, punctuation and abbreviations, presentation of numbers and statistics, construction of tables and

figures, citation of references, and many other elements that are a part of a manuscript.

- *Vancouver style:* Vancouver is a generic term for a style of referencing widely used in the health sciences, using a numbered reference list. There is no official manual of the Vancouver style, but the United States National Library of Medicine's style guide is now considered the most authoritative manual on this type of referencing.

- *Modern Language Association (MLA) citation style:* The MLA system uses in-text citations rather than footnotes or endnotes. The citations in-text are very brief, usually just the author's family name and a relevant page number.

- *The Chicago manual of style:* The Chicago manual of style is the most widely consulted of all style manuals. It includes provisions for footnote referencing and author-date referencing. The Chicago manual's footnote referencing system is widely used in the arts and humanities.

### *Examples*

| Style of citation | Example |
| --- | --- |
| MLA | Lozhkin, Andrey, et al. "NADPH oxidase 4 regulates vascular inflammation in aging and atherosclerosis." Journal of Molecular and Cellular Cardiology 102 (2017): 10–21. |
| APA | Lozhkin, A, Vendrov, AE, Pan, H, Wickline, SA, Madamanchi, NR, and Runge, MS (2017). NADPH oxidase 4 regulates vascular inflammation in aging and atherosclerosis. Journal of Molecular and Cellular Cardiology, 102, 10–21. |
| Chicago | Lozhkin, Andrey, Aleksandr E. Vendrov, Hua Pan, Samuel A. Wickline, Nageswara R. Madamanchi, and Marschall S. Runge. "NADPH oxidase 4 regulates vascular inflammation in aging and atherosclerosis." Journal of Molecular and Cellular Cardiology 102 (2017): 10–21. |
| Harvard | Lozhkin, A, Vendrov, AE, Pan, H, Wickline, SA, Madamanchi, NR and Runge, MS, 2017. NADPH oxidase 4 regulates vascular inflammation in aging and atherosclerosis. Journal of Molecular and Cellular Cardiology, 102, pp.10–21. |
| Vancouver | Lozhkin A, Vendrov AE, Pan H, Wickline SA, Madamanchi NR, Runge MS. NADPH oxidase 4 regulates vascular inflammation in aging and atherosclerosis. Journal of Molecular and Cellular Cardiology. 2017 Jan 31;102:10–21. |

**Science citation index:** A citation index is a kind of bibliographic index, an index of citations between publications, allowing the user to easily establish which later documents cite earlier documents. A form of citation index is first found in 12th-century Hebrew religious literature. Legal citation indexes are found in the 18th century and were made popular by citators such as Shepard's Citations (1873). In 1960, Eugene Garfield's Institute for Scientific Information (ISI) introduced the first citation index for papers published in academic journals, first the science citation index (SCI), and later the social sciences citation index (SSCI) and the arts and humanities citation index (AHCI). The first automated citation indexing was done by CiteSeer in 1997. Other sources for such data include general purpose academic citation indexes include:

- Web of Science by Clarivate Analytics (previously the Intellectual Property and Science business of Thomson Reuters).
- Scopus by Elsevier available online only, which similarly combines subject searching with citation browsing and tracking in the sciences and social sciences.
- Indian citation index is an online citation data which covers peer reviewed journals published from India. It covers major subject areas such as scientific, technical, medical, and social sciences and includes arts and humanities. The citation database is the first of its kind in India.

## Bibliography

1. Coventry University Harvard Reference Style Guide By Lisa Ganobcsik Williams and Catalina Neculai, Pg. No. 7.
2. Curtis, MJ, Bond, RA, Spina, D, Ahluwalia, A, Alexander, S, Giembycz, MA, and Lawrence, AJ (2015). Experimental design and analysis and their reporting: new guidance for publication in BJP. British journal of pharmacology, 172(14), 3461–3471.
3. Ghosh, M (2007). Fundamentals of experimental pharmacology. Indian Journal of Pharmacology, 39(4), 216–216.
4. Library Services Help Sheet, London South Bank University, Perry Library and Learning Resources Pg. No. 2.

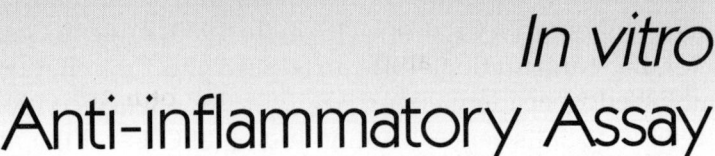

# CHAPTER 2

# *In vitro* Anti-inflammatory Assay

**Inflammation** is the reaction of living tissues to injury, infection or irritation.

**Inflammation versus infection:** Infection is the consequence of invasion of a foreign pathogen such as a virus, a bacterium, or a fungus in a healthy human body. On the other hand, inflammation is the body's immune response to a pathogen or an invader. The body sends white blood cells (pus) to fight off the infection, and chemicals are released that cause the classic symptoms of inflammation.

**Types:** Inflammation can be classified as either acute or chronic.

- *Acute inflammation* is the initial response of the body to harmful stimuli and is achieved by the increased movement of plasma and leukocytes (especially granulocytes) from the blood into the injured tissues. A series of biochemical events propagates and matures the inflammatory response, involving the local vascular system, the immune system, and various cells within the injured tissue.

- *Chronic inflammation* or prolonged inflammation which leads to a progressive shift in the type of cells present at the site of inflammation, such as mononuclear cells, and is characterized by simultaneous destruction and healing of the tissue from the inflammatory process.

**Symptoms:** The classic signs of inflammation are heat, redness, swelling, pain, and loss of function.

## Mediators of Inflammation

- *Physical agents*: Extreme temperatures, electric shock, radiation, and mechanical injures.
- *Chemical agents*: Products of metabolism, acids, alkalis, drugs and conditions leading to tissue necrosis.

- *Biological agents*: Microorganisms (bacteria, viruses, fungi), parasites (helminths, insects), immune cells and complexes.

**Pathophysiology:** These are manifestations of the physiologic changes that occur during the inflammatory process. The three major components of this process are:

- Hemodynamic changes that begin soon after injury and progress at varying rates, according to the extent of injury. They start with dilation of the arterioles and the opening of new capillaries and venular beds in the area. This causes an accelerated flow of blood, accounting for the signs of heat and redness.

- Increased capillary permeability permits leakage of protein-rich fluid out of small blood vessels and into the extravascular fluid compartment, accounting for the inflammatory edema.

- Leukocytic exudation involves the movement of the leukocytes to the endothelial lining of the small blood vessels. Eventually, these leukocytes move through the endothelial spaces and escape into the extravascular space. Once they are outside the blood vessels they are free to move and, by chemotaxis, are drawn to the site of injury. Accumulations of neutrophils and macrophages at the area of inflammation act to neutralize foreign particles by phagocytosis.

**Physiological significance of inflammation:** Inflammation is exceedingly complex and equally fascinating. It has a crucial role in mammalian physiology. The effectors of an inflammatory response are the tissues and cells, the functional states of which are specifically affected by the inflammatory mediators. Although the most obvious effect of inflammatory mediators is to induce the formation of an exudate, many inflammatory mediators have other, equally important, effects on neuroendocrine and metabolic functions and on the maintenance of tissue homeostasis in general. These functions of inflammatory mediators reflect a more general role for inflammation in the control of tissue homeostasis and in adaptation to noxious conditions. Homeostatic control mechanisms ensure that internal environmental parameters (such as glucose and oxygen concentrations) are maintained within an acceptable range. Abnormal conditions can cause a deviation in some parameters beyond the normal homeostatic range, resulting in a more sustained adaptive change that involves a shift in the relevant set points. In a general sense, acute inflammation and chronic inflammation are different types of adaptive response that are called into action when other homeostatic mechanisms are either insufficient or not competent. The inflammatory response is commonly thought to operate during severe disturbances of homeostasis, such as infection and injury. Whatever the cause of the inflammatory response, its 'purpose' is to remove or sequester the source of the disturbance, to allow the host to adapt to the abnormal conditions and, ultimately, to restore functionality and homeostasis to the tissue.

**Pathological consequences of inflammation:** Inflammatory diseases include a vast array of disorders and conditions that are as pathological consequence of inflammation. Examples include allergy, asthma, autoimmune diseases, coeliac disease, glomerulonephritis, hepatitis, inflammatory bowel disease, preperfusion injury and transplant rejection. Inflammatory processes may also play a critical role in the degeneration of basal forebrain cholinergic cells that underlie some of the degenerative disorders like the Alzheimer's disease.

## Bibliography

1. Coussens, LM, and Werb, Z (2002). Inflammation and cancer. Nature, 420(6917), 860–867.
2. Dai, X and Medzhitov, R (2017). Inflammation: Memory beyond immunity. Nature, 550(7677), 460.

## EXPERIMENT 2.1

**Aim:** To study the *in vitro* anti-inflammatory potential of the given sample against heat-induced protein denaturation.

**Principle:** Protein denaturation is a process in which proteins lose their tertiary structure and secondary structure by application of external stress or compounds, such as strong acid or base, a concentrated inorganic salt, an organic solvent or heat. Most biological proteins lose their biological function when denatured. Denaturation of protein is a well-documented cause of inflammation.

## Requirements

*Chemicals*: Standard drug solution (aspirin or diclofenac), test sample solution, egg albumin or 1% bovine serum albumin (BSA) solution, phosphate buffered saline and 1N hydrochloric acid solution.

*Equipment*: UV-visible spectrophotometer, incubator and water bath.

*Glasswares*: Beakers, pipettes, measuring cylinder and glass rod.

## Procedure

1. Prepare 1% solution of BSA or 1 mM egg albumin solution.
2. Prepare 5 mL reaction mixture by adding 0.2 mL of egg albumin (or 1% BSA solution), 2.8 mL phosphate buffered saline (pH 6.4) and 2 mL of varying concentration of sample solution.
3. Incubate the reaction mixture at 37±2°C in an incubator for 15 minutes and then denaturation is induced by keeping the reaction mixture at 70°C in a water bath for 10 minutes.
4. After cooling, measure absorbance at 660 nm by spectrophotometer using vehicle as blank.
5. Similar reaction mixture composed of similar volume of double distilled water instead of test sample serve as control.
6. Diclofenac at the final concentration of (1 mg/mL) is used as reference drug and treated similarly for determination of absorbance.
7. The experiment is performed in triplicates.
8. Record the absorbances and calculate percentage inhibition of both test and standard according to the prescribed formula.

## Observation

| S. no. | Absorbance of control | Absorbance of test | Absorbance of standard |
|--------|----------------------|-------------------|------------------------|
| 1. | | | |
| 2. | | | |
| 3. | | | |

**Calculation:** The percentage inhibition of protein denaturation was calculated as follows:

$$\text{Percentage inhibition} = \frac{(\text{Abs control} - \text{Abs sample})}{\text{Abs control}} \times 100$$

where, Abs control—absorbance of control (the control represents 100% protein denaturation)

Abs sample—absorbance of sample

## Bibliography

1. Ingle, PV, and Patel, DM (2011). C-reactive protein in various disease condition-an overview. Asian J Pharm Clin Res, 4(1), 9–13.
2. Shipton, FN, Khoo, TJ, Hossan, MS, and Wiart, C (2017). Activity of Pericampylus glaucus and periglaucine A *in vitro* against nasopharangeal carcinoma and anti-inflammatory activity. Journal of ethnopharmacology, 198, 91–97.

**Aim:** To study the *in vitro* anti-inflammatory potential of the given sample by membrane stabilization assay (heat-induced hemolysis).

**Principle:** Neutrophils and macrophages at the area of inflammation act to neutralize foreign particles by phagocytosis. These phagocytic cells use reactive oxygen species in combination with proteases to destroy ingested foreign particles. The reactive oxygen species, however, elicits lipid peroxidation and membrane destabilization, thereby increasing mucosal permeability in inflamed tissue. In membrane stabilization method, absorbance of hemoglobin is determined. The hemoglobin is released as a result of lyses of RBC membrane, due to less stabilization of membrane.

## Requirements

*Chemicals*: Standard drug solution (aspirin or diclofenac), test sample solution, whole human blood, isotonic buffered solution (154 mM NaCl) in 10 mM sodium phosphate buffer (pH 7.4), and normal saline solution.

*Equipment*: UV-visible spectrophotometer, incubator and heating mantle.

*Glasswares*: Beakers, pipettes, measuring cylinder and glass rod.

## Procedure

1. Collect approximately 5.0 mL human blood in heparinized centrifuge tube from healthy human volunteers who has not taken any non-steroidal anti-inflammatory drug (NSAID) for 2 weeks prior to the experiment or animal sample acquired from animal model.

2. Prepare human red blood cells (HRBC) or erythrocyte suspension by washing and centrifuging the collected blood with isotonic buffer solution (10 mM sodium phosphate buffer with 7.4 pH) for 10 minutes at 3,000 rpm. Carefully pipette out the supernatant and re-suspended the packed cells with equal volume of buffer solution (pH 7.4) and centrifuge again. Repeat the process until a clear supernatant is obtained. A 10% HRBC suspension is then prepared with normal saline and used immediately.

3. Prepare reaction mixture by adding 0.5 mL of 10% HRBC suspension in 3.5 mL of sodium phosphate buffer (pH 7.4) and then add 1 mL of test sample dissolved in normal physiological saline.

4. Incubate the reaction mixture at 37°C for 15 minutes.

5. Perform two controls, one with 1.0 mL of isotonic saline instead of extract and the second control with 0.5 mL of isotonic saline instead of red blood cells.

6. Incubate the mixture in a water bath at 56°C for 30 minutes. Cool the tubes under running water for 20 minutes.

7. After cooling, absorbance is measured at 560 nm by using vehicle as blank.

8. Diclofenac at the final concentration of 1 mg/mL is used as reference drug and treated similarly for determination of absorbance.

9. The experiment is performed in triplicates.

10. Record the absorbances and calculate percentage inhibition of hemolysis for both test and standard according to the prescribed formula.

## Observation

| S. no. | Absorbance of control | Absorbance of test | Absorbance of standard |
|--------|----------------------|--------------------|------------------------|
| 1. | | | |
| 2. | | | |
| 3. | | | |

**Calculation:** The percentage inhibition of hemolysis can be calculated as follows:

$$\text{Percentage inhibition of hemolysis} = \frac{(\text{Abs control} - \text{Abs sample})}{\text{Abs control}} \times 100$$

where,  Abs control—absorbance of control (the control represents 100% protein denaturation)

Abs sample—absorbance of sample

## Bibliography

1. Chen, GY, and Nuñez, G (2010). Sterile inflammation: sensing and reacting to damage. Nature Reviews. Immunology, 10(12), 826–837.

2. Tantary, S, Masood, A, Bhat, AH, Dar, KB, Zargar, MA, and Ganie, SA (2017). *In vitro* Antioxidant and RBC membrane Stabilization Activity of *Euphorbia wallichii*. Free Radicals and Antioxidants, 7(1), 13.

## EXPERIMENT 2.3

**Aim:** To study the *in vitro* anti-inflammatory potential of the given sample by membrane stabilization assay (hypotonicity-induced hemolysis).

**Principle:** Neutrophils and macrophages at the area of inflammation act to neutralize foreign particles by phagocytosis. These phagocytic cells use reactive oxygen species in combination with proteases to destroy ingested foreign particles. The reactive oxygen species, however, elicits lipid peroxidation and membrane destabilization, thereby increasing mucosal permeability in inflamed tissue. In membrane stabilization method, absorbance of hemoglobin is determined. The hemoglobin is released as a result of lyses of RBC membrane, due to less stabilization of membrane.

## Requirements

*Chemicals*: Standard drug solution (aspirin or diclofenac), test sample solution, whole human blood, isotonic buffered solution (154 mM NaCl) in 10 mM sodium phosphate buffer (pH 7.4), and normal saline solution.

*Equipment*: UV-visible spectrophotometer, incubator and heating mantle.

*Glasswares*: Beakers, pipettes, measuring cylinder and glass rod.

## Procedure

1. Collect approximately 5.0 mL of whole human blood in heparinized centrifuge tube from healthy human volunteer who has not taken any NSAID for 2 weeks prior to the experiment.
2. Prepare human red blood cells (HRBC) solution by washing and centrifuging the collected blood with isotonic buffered solution (154 mM NaCl) in 10 mM sodium phosphate buffer (pH 7.4) for 10 minutes at 3,000 rpm. Carefully pipette out the supernatant. Resuspend the packed cells with equal volume of normal saline (pH 7.4) and centrifuge again. Repeat the process until clear supernatants is obtained. A 10% HRBC suspension is then prepared with normal saline and use immediately.
3. Prepare 4.5 mL of reaction mixture consisting of 2 mL hypotonic saline, 1 mL of sodium phosphate buffer (0.15 M, pH 7.4) and 1 mL of sample is dissolved in normal physiological saline. Then add 0.5 mL of 10% HRBC.
4. Perform two controls, one with 1.0 mL of isotonic saline instead of extract and the second control with 0.5 mL of isotonic saline instead of red blood cells.

5. Incubate the mixture at 37°C for 30 minutes. Cool the tubes under running water for 20 minutes.
6. After cooling, measure absorbance 560 nm by using vehicle as blank.
7. Diclofenac at the final concentration of 1 mg/mL is used as reference drug and treated similarly for determination of absorbance.
8. The experiment is performed in triplicates.
9. Record the absorbances and calculate percentage inhibition of hemolysis for both test and standard according to the prescribed formula.

## Observation

| S. no. | Absorbance of control | Absorbance of test | Absorbance of standard |
|--------|-----------------------|--------------------|------------------------|
| 1. | | | |
| 2. | | | |
| 3. | | | |

**Calculation:** The percentage inhibition of hemolysis can be calculated as follows:

$$\text{Percentage inhibition of hemolysis} = \frac{(\text{Abs control} - \text{Abs sample})}{\text{Abs control}} \times 100$$

where,   Abs control—absorbance of control (the control represents 100% hemolysis)

Abs sample—absorbance of sample

## Bibliography

1. Chen, GY, and Nuñez, G (2010). Sterile inflammation: sensing and reacting to damage. Nature Reviews. Immunology, 10(12), 826–837.
2. Tantary, S, Masood, A, Bhat, AH, Dar, KB, Zargar, MA, and Ganie, SA (2017). *In vitro* Antioxidant and RBC membrane Stabilization Activity of *Euphorbia wallichii*. Free Radicals and Antioxidants, 7(1), 13.

**EXPERIMENT 2.4**

**Aim:** To study the *in vitro* 5-lipoxygenase inhibitory potential of the given sample using 5-lipoxygenase inhibition assay.

**Principle:** The mammalian enzyme 5-lipoxygenase plays an important role in the conversion of arachidonic acid to a number of lipoxygenase derivatives, including 5-HPETE, $LTA_4$, $LTB_4$ and peptidoleukotrienes $LTC_4$, $LTD_4$ and $LTE_4$. The leukotrienes have been identified as a component of SRS-A (slow-reacting substance of anaphylaxis). Since these mediators have been demonstrated to possess potent chemotactic, bronchoconstrictor, and vascular leakage properties. They have also been implicated as important mediators of various allergic diseases including asthma. Various lipoxygenase products ($LTB_4$) also exhibit proinflammatory properties both *in vitro* and *in vivo*. Thus inhibition of 5-lipoxygenase is currently a subject of intense research targeted towards the discovery of novel anti-allergic and anti-inflammatory agents.

Lipoxygenases catalyse the reaction of polyenoic fatty acids, containing at least 1,4-*cis* or *cis*-pentadiene system, with dioxygen forming a 1-hydroperoxy-2-*trans*, 4-*cis* derivative. 5-Lipoxygenase inhibition activity is measured by the increase in absorbance at 234 nm following incubation of the enzyme with the substrate.

## Requirements

*Chemicals*: Test sample, hyaluronidase enzyme, phosphate buffer (pH 7), calcium chloride ($CaCl_2$), potassium hyaluronate, potassium tetraborate, sodium hydroxide (NaOH) and *p*-DMAB.

*Equipment*: UV-visible spectrophotometer.

*Glasswares*: Test tubes, micropipettes, measuring cylinder and glass rod.

## Procedure

1. Put 0.95 mL of 0.1 M phosphate buffer, pH 7.4, in precooled quartz cuvette.
2. Prepare lipoxygenase enzyme solution such that the enzyme concentration in the reaction mixture is adjusted to give a rate of 0.05 absorbance per minutes.
3. Add the enzyme solution.
4. Prepare test sample solution by dissolving test sample in methanol, ethanol, 2-methoxy ethanol (methyl glycol) or DMSO as 0.1 M solution. Add the test sample solution in the proper dilution in the same solvent

in such a volume that the final concentration of the solvent does not exceed 2% of final volume. Add the same amount of solvent to identically handled control samples.

5. Add about 50 µL of the solution of test compound. Incubate for 5–10 minutes at 20°C.

6. Start the reaction by adding 50 µL of substrate mixture. Prepare substrate mixture by mixing 0.2 mL of pure linoleic acid (or arachidonic acid) with 1 mL of freshly distilled methanol. Store this stock solution under nitrogen atmosphere at –20°C. Mix 20 mL of the stock solution with 20 mL of 0.54 M KOH or 0.54 M NH$_4$OH. Add this freshly prepared mixture to 2 mL of cold 0.1 M phosphate buffer.

7. Mix gently and record the absorbance at 234 nm for 2–3 minutes.

## Observation

| S. no. | Absorbance of control | Absorbance of test | Absorbance of standard |
|--------|----------------------|--------------------|------------------------|
| 1. | | | |
| 2. | | | |
| 3. | | | |

**Calculation:** The percentage inhibition of enzyme is calculated as follows:

$$\% \text{ inhibition of 5-lipoxygenase} = \frac{(\text{Abs control} - \text{Abs sample})}{\text{Abs control}} \times 100$$

where,  Abs control—absorbance of control

Abs sample—absorbance of sample

## Bibliography

1. Kretschmer, SB, Woltersdorf, S, Vogt, D, Lillich, FF, Rühl, M, Karas, M, and Wurglics, M (2017). Characterization of the molecular mechanism of 5-lipoxygenase inhibition by 2-aminothiazoles. Biochemical pharmacology, 123, 52–62.

2. Maucher, IV, Rühl, M, Kretschmer, SB, Hofmann, B, Kühn, B, Fettel, J, and Häfner, AK (2017). Michael acceptor containing drugs are a novel class of 5-lipoxygenase inhibitor targeting the surface cysteines C416 and C418. Biochemical Pharmacology, 125, 55–74.

## EXPERIMENT 2.5

**Aim:** To study the *in vitro* hyaluronidase inhibitory potential of the given sample using hyaluronidase inhibition assay.

**Principle:** Hyaluronidase, a mucopolysaccharide hydrolyzing enzyme, has been shown to involve in various diseases. The enzyme is functionally related to vascular permeability and inflammatory reactions. Since the enzyme exists in an inactive form, its *in vivo* activation by metal ions including calcium ions is related to the degranulation of mast cells, causing release of mediators that cause allergy including inflammation. Hyaluronate, a mucopolysaccaharide, consisting of repeating subunits of D-glucuronic acid and N-acetyl-D-glucosamine, is a viscous lubricating agent present in synovial fluid in joints. In rheumatoid arthritis, its excessive degradation by hyaluronidase may lead to decrease in amount and molecular weight of hyaluronate thus producing arthritic symptoms. The search for inhibitors of hyaluronidase enzyme may lead to the isolation of new potent anti-allergic and anti-inflammatory drugs.

Hyaluronidase enzyme hydrolytically cleaves the (1–4) bond in hyaluronic acid liberating the product with a terminal N-acetyl-D-glucosamine moiety that reacts with alkali to form a glucoxazoline an intermediate compound. This intermediate reacts with *p*-dimethylaminobenzaldehyde (*p*-DMAB) to produce a colored product which is measured at 585 nm.

### Requirements

*Chemicals:* Test sample, hyaluronidase enzyme, phosphate buffer (pH 7), calcium chloride ($CaCl_2$), potassium hyaluronate, potassium tetraborate, sodium hydroxide (NaOH) and *p*-DMAB.

*Equipment:* UV-visible spectrophotometer.

*Glasswares:* Test tubes, micropipettes, measuring cylinder and glass rod.

### Procedure

*a. Activation of Hyaluronidase Enzyme*

1. Take 400 µL of hyaluronidase enzyme solution (350 N.F. units/mL of acetate buffer) in a screw cap test tube.
2. Add 100 µL of $CaCl_2$ solution (2.5 mM in acetate buffer) to this test tube and incubated at 37°C for 20 minutes to activate the enzyme.

### b. Inhibition of Activated Hyaluronidase Enzyme

1. Add 100 μL of test sample or vehicle to the activated enzyme. This mixture is incubated at 37°C for 20 minutes in a water bath.
2. Add 500 μL of potassium hyaluronate (1.2 mg/mL of acetate buffer) and carry out incubation again at 37°C for 20 minutes.
3. Stop the enzyme reaction by adding 100 μL of NaOH (0.4 N) and 100 μL of potassium tetraborate (0.8 N, pH 9.1).
4. Heat the mixture in a boiling water bath for exactly 3 minutes and cool the tubes with tap water.
5. Add 3 mL of *p*-DMAB solution (67 mM) mix and incubate at 37°C for 20 minutes for color development.
6. The absorbance of the mixture is measured at 585 nm in a spectrophotometer against blank.

### c. Inhibition of the Activation of Inactive Hyaluronidase Enzyme

1. Take 400 μL of hyaluronidase enzyme solution (350 N.F. units/mL of acetate buffer) in a screw cap test tube.
2. Add 100 μL of test sample or vehicle mixed and incubated at 37°C for 20 minutes.
3. Add 100 μL of CaCl$_2$ (2.5 mM in acetate buffer) added and incubated at 37°C for 20 minutes.
4. Repeat the procedure described from step 3 onward in protocol *b*.

### Observation

| S. no. | Absorbance of control | Absorbance of test | Absorbance of standard |
|--------|----------------------|--------------------|------------------------|
| 1. | | | |
| 2. | | | |
| 3. | | | |

**Calculation:** The percentage inhibition of hyaluronidase is calculated as follows:

$$\% \text{ inhibition of hyaluronidase} = \frac{(\text{Abs control} - \text{Abs sample})}{\text{Abs control}} \times 100$$

where,  Abs control—absorbance of control
      Abs sample—absorbance of sample

## Bibliography

1. Druker, BJ, Tamura, S, Buchdunger, E, Ohno, S, Segal, GM, Fanning, S, and Lydon, NB (1996). Effects of a selective inhibitor of the Abl tyrosine kinase on the growth of Bcr-Abl positive cells. Nature Medicine, 2(5), 561–566.

2. Rusnak, DW, Lackey, K, Affleck, K, Wood, ER, Alligood, KJ, Rhodes, N, and Gilmer, TM (2001). The effects of the novel, reversible epidermal growth factor receptor/ ErbB-2 tyrosine kinase inhibitor, GW2016, on the growth of human normal and tumor-derived cell lines *in vitro* and *in vivo*. Molecular Cancer Therapeutics, 1(2), 85–94.

## *IN VITRO* CYCLO-OXYGENASE ENZYME ASSAY

Cyclo-oxygenase (COX, also known as prostaglandin G/H synthase) is a membrane bound enzyme responsible for the oxidation of arachidonic acid to prostaglandin G (PGG) and the subsequent reduction of PGG to PGH (Fig. 2.1). These reactions result in the formation of a variety of prostanoids. COX has been shown to be expressed in at least two different isoforms, i.e. a constitutively expressed form, COX-I, and an inducible form, COX-II. COX-I is thought to regulate a number of 'housekeeping' functions, such as vascular hemostasis, renal blood flow, and maintenance of glomerular function. Inflammation mediators such as growth factors, cytokines and endotoxin induce COX-II expression in a number of cellular systems. The effect of various non-steroidal anti-inflammatory drugs (NSAIDs) on the activity of COX-I and -II is an area of considerable interest. Some methods to determine COX activity involve procedures such as measuring uptake of oxygen using an oxygraph, measuring the conversion of radioactive arachidonic acid, or measuring the prostaglandins formed from PGH (such as determining PGE using immunoassays. Most of these methods are complex, time consuming, and are prone to interferences. However, determination of COX inhibitory potential is most important parameter in defining the anti-inflammatory property of any new drug entity.

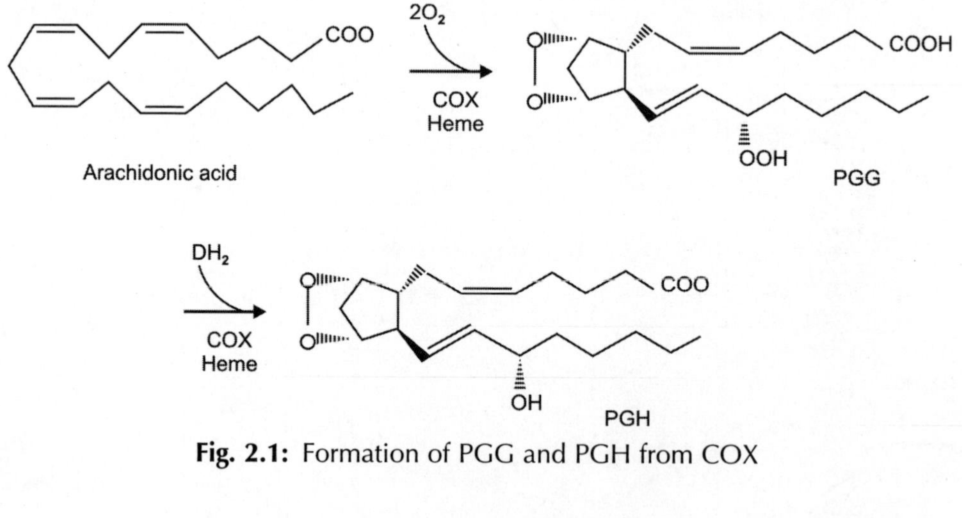

**Fig. 2.1:** Formation of PGG and PGH from COX

## EXPERIMENT 2.6

**Aim:** To study the *in vitro* anti-inflammatory potential of the given sample by COX inhibition using luminescent assay protocol.

**Principle:** The COX activity by luminescent assay uses a specific chemiluminescent substrate to detect the peroxidative activity of COX enzymes. After inhibition by NSAIDs, the direct residual activity of COX is measured by addition of a proprietary luminescent substrate and arachidonic acid. Light emission starts immediately and is directly proportional to the COX activity in the sample. The chemiluminescent signals are measured over 5 seconds.

### Requirements

*Chemicals:* Standard drug solution (ibuprofen or meloxicam), test sample solution, deionized or distilled water, and COX enzyme assay kit.

*Equipment:* White 96-well microtiter plate, plate luminometer with dual injectors incubator and water bath.

*Glasswares:* Beakers, pipettes, measuring cylinder and glass rod.

### Procedure

1. *Reagent Preparation Method*
   i. Store COX-I and/or COX-II at −70°C or lower. Enzyme dilutions in 100 mM phosphate, pH 7.5, used for inhibition reactions, must be kept at 0–4°C in an ice bath. These enzyme dilutions are stable for 2–8 hours.
   ii. Prepare hematin (porcine) by dissolving in DMSO at 0.38 mg/mL. The concentrated stock can be stored at −80°C in single use volumes. Dilute in 100 mM phosphate, pH 7.5 to a final concentration of 0.12 µM. Diluted hematin is stable for up to 8 hours at room temperature.

**Note:** Avoid exposure to light. Higher concentrations of hematin give rise to increasing background signals and do not result in increased cyclooxygenase actvity or increased inhibition by NSAIDs.

   iii. Prepare a 100 mM Tris, 0.5 mM phenol buffer, pH 7.3 buffer pH must be measured at 37°C for correct pH measurement.
   iv. Arachidonic acid stock solution in ethanol is prepared by taking a freshly opened vial of arachidonic acid and adding ethanol under argon or nitrogen gas to give a 50 mg/mL solution. Store in the dark at −70°C or lower.

v. Activation of arachadonic acid is carried out by the following procedure. Add 94 µL of 0.1 N sodium hydroxide to a glass vial. Add 6 µL of the ethanolic arachadonic acid solution to the vial. Vortex the reaction mixture. Dilute the mixture with 9.9 mL of deionized water. Store the prepared solution of arachidonic acid at 0–4°C in an ice bath; it is stable for up to 3 hours.

**Note:** For best reproducibility store the prepared arachadonic acid solution at 0–4°C in the luminometer. Injection of the cold arachadonic acid solution is recommended.

### 2. Assay Protocol

i. Do not mix reagents from different lot numbers. Allow all reagents to warm to room temperature for at least 30 minutes before opening. Prerinse the pipette tip with reagent, use fresh pipet tips for each sample, standard and reagent.

ii. Add the reagents to the side of the well to avoid contamination. Mix the substrate well prior to use. Pipet 50 µL of the Tris-phenol buffer into all wells. Add 50 µL of the hematin solution into all wells.

iii. Add 50 µL COX-I or COX-II preparations to all wells, except for the blank and zero activity wells.

iv. Pre-incubate at room temperature for 5 minutes. Add 25 µL of NSAID inhibitor solution to appropriate wells.

v. Incubate at room temperature for 5–120 minutes (dependent on inhibitor).

vi. Place microtiter plate in luminometer for the chemiluminescent measurement.

vii. Inject 50 µL of cold COX chemiluminescent substrate. Immediately inject 50 µL of diluted cold arachidonic acid solution.

viii. Immediately read in a luminometer for 5 seconds. Determine integrated light output for the 5-second read time in relative light units (RLU).

### Observation

| S. no. | RLU of blank | RLU of test | RLU of standard |
|---|---|---|---|
| 1. | | | |
| 2. | | | |
| 3. | | | |

**Calculation:** The percentage COX inhibition can be calculated as follows:

$$\text{Percentage inhibition} = 1-\left(\frac{\text{RLU}_{AN}}{\text{RLU}_{AN}-\text{for noninhibited}}\right)\times100$$

where, RLU—relative light unit

RLU$_{AN}$—average net inhibitor (RLU)

RLU$_{AN}$—average RLU − Average blank RLU

**Note:** One unit of COX activity is defined as the amount of enzyme needed to consume 1 nmole of oxygen per minute at 37°C.

## Bibliography

1. Hasinoff, BB, Patel, D, and Wu, X (2007). The cytotoxicity of celecoxib towards cardiac myocytes is cyclooxygenase-2 independent. Cardiovascular Toxicology, 7(1), 19–27.

2. Nikolic, D, Habibi-Goudarzi, S, Corley, DG, Gafner, S, Pezzuto, JM, and Van Breemen, RB (2000). Evaluation of cyclooxygenase-2 inhibitors using pulsed ultrafiltration mass spectrometry. Analytical Chemistry, 72(16), 3853–3859.

## EXPERIMENT 2.7

**Aim:** To study the *in vitro* COX inhibition potential of the given sample by using oxygen uptake assay protocol.

**Principle:** The conversion of arachidonic acid to the unstable hydroperoxide intermediate $PGG_2$ can be monitored directly by measuring the oxygen consumed during the reaction using an oxygen sensor. The reaction requires two moles of molecular oxygen per mole of arachidonic acid. Since most NSAIDs inhibit the cyclo-oxygenase activity of COX, but not the peroxidase activity, this assay can serve as a direct measure of inhibition. Initial rates of the reaction can be quantified, which is essential for determining the properties of competitive inhibitors.

### Requirements

*Chemicals:* Tris/heme/phenol (THP) buffer, sodium dithionite, saturated solution 2 mg/mL cyclo-oxygenase (COX) enzyme solution (20–30 µg per reaction) inhibitors dissolved in dimethylsulfoxide (DMSO), 10 mM arachidonic acid, methanol.

*Equipment:* Clark-style polarographic electrode, with 600 µL water-jacketed reaction vessel, chart recorder (2 V full-scale input) or IBM-compatible computer with intake software, 37°C recirculating water bath, two peristaltic pumps.

*Glasswares:* Two 10 µL and one 50 µL Hamilton syringes, four-way valve, beakers, pipettes, measuring cylinder and glass rod.

### Procedure

1. Prepare 200 mL THP buffer and place it in a flask in a 37°C recirculating water bath 1 hour prior to assay to ensure proper oxygen saturation of the reagent solution and thermal equilibration of the assay vessel. While the reagent is equilibrating, prepare the Clark-style polarographic electrode according to the manufacturer's instructions and set up the 600 µL water-jacketed reaction vessel.

2. Activate oxygen sensor amplifiers and calibrate the system as directed by the manufacturer. Adjust chart recorder by setting the full-scale pen deflection at 100% oxygen saturation (~217 µM at 37°C). Zero the system with a saturated solution of sodium dithionite.

3. Once the system has stabilized, add THP buffer to the reaction vessel with a peristaltic pump at a flow rate of ~2 mL/min, for 30 seconds. Add

10 µL of 2 mg/mL COX enzyme solution (20 µg, 460 nM) with a 10 µL Hamilton syringe to the top fill port. Incubate 30 seconds to reconstitute the enzyme with heme.

4. Add 6 µL inhibitor or DMSO solvent to the top fill port using a Hamilton syringe. Incubate for various amounts of time, depending on the application.

   *Recommended incubation time is 2 seconds to 5 minutes. In cases where enzyme is added to initiate the reaction (competitive kinetics), this step should be performed first and enzyme should be reconstituted with heme prior to addition.*

5. Activate the chart recorder and initiate the reaction by adding 6 µL of 10 mM arachidonic acid (100 µM final). The reaction is essentially complete after 30 seconds.

6. Turn the four-way valve to the rinse solution and rinse the reaction vessel for 2 minutes with either $H_2O$ or methanol. During the rinse, data from the run can be analyzed and the data system reset for the next run.

7. Calculate activity in terms of micromoles $O_2$ consumed per minute at maximal velocity.

   *The Instech system is connected to an IBM-compatible computer, and the Intake software automatically provides the instantaneous velocity, in micromoles $O_2$ consumed per minute, at any point.*

8. Enzyme activity can also be determined manually with a chart recorder by drawing a tangential line to the plot at its steepest point, which is linear for the first ~10 sec. A full-scale deflection represents consumption of 0.139 mol $O_2$. Convert the rate of $O_2$ consumed per minute to enzyme units using this value and the chart speed of the recorder.

## Observation

| S. no. | Oxygen consumed | | |
|--------|-----------------|------|----------|
|        | Control | Test | Standard |
| 1.     |         |      |          |
| 2.     |         |      |          |
| 3.     |         |      |          |

**Calculation:** The percentage COX inhibition can be calculated as follows:

$$\text{Percentage inhibition} = \left( \frac{O_c - O_T}{O_c} \right) \times 100$$

where,   $O_c$—oxygen consumption by control
$O_T$—oxygen consumption by test

**Note:** One unit of COX activity is defined as the amount of enzyme needed to consume 1 nmole of oxygen per minute at 37°C.

## Bibliography

1. Mashhadi, Z, Boeglin, WE, and Brash, AR (2015). Robust inhibitory effects of conjugated linolenic acids on a cyclooxygenase-related linoleate 10S-dioxygenase: comparison with COX-1 and COX-2. Biochimica et Biophysica Acta (BBA)-Molecular and Cell Biology of Lipids, 1851(10), 1346–1352.
2. Ratchford, SM, Lavin, KM, Perkins, RK, Jemiolo, B, Trappe, SW, and Trappe, TA (2017). Aspirin as a COX inhibitor and anti-inflammatory drug in human skeletal muscle. Journal of Applied Physiology, 123(6), 1610–1616.

## EXPERIMENT 2.8

**Aim:** To study the *in vitro* COX inhibition potential of the given sample by using peroxidase assay.

**Principle:** The activity of COX is measured here by utilizing its intrinsic peroxidase activity and the electron donor TMPD, which turns blue upon reduction, as a cosubstrate. TMPD will not turn over without the presence of a hydroperoxide substrate. In this case either arachidonic acid (which forms a hydroperoxide in the presence of COX) or hydrogen peroxide can be used as a substrate. By using hydrogen peroxide, it is possible to directly measure peroxidase activity; with arachidonic acid, which must first be converted to a hydroperoxide, the assay yields an indirect measure of COX activity.

### Requirements

*Chemicals:* Peroxidase assay buffer, 2 mg/mL cyclo-oxygenase (COX) enzyme solution, inhibitors, dissolved in dimethylsulfoxide (DMSO), N, N, N′, N′-tetramethyl-*p*-phenylenediamine (N, N′N′-TMPD), and 10 mM arachidonic acid.

*Equipment:* Visible spectrophotometer or 96-well plate reader with 590–611 nm filter.

*Glasswares:* Beakers, pipettes, measuring cylinder and glass rod.

### Procedure

1. Add 960 µL peroxidase assay buffer to a single 1 cm disposable plastic cuvette. Add 10 µL of 2 mg/mL COX enzyme solution and let the enzyme equilibrate ~30 seconds with the heme in the assay buffer.

2. For kinetic analysis, add the enzyme last, in which case the enzyme should be reconstituted with heme before use (1 M heme, 5 minutes). The amount of enzyme can be varied depending on purity. Reactions can be performed at room temperature.

3. Add 10 µL inhibitor or DMSO solvent for various amounts of time (e.g. 2 seconds to 5 minutes).

4. Initiate the reaction by adding 10 µL of 17 mM TMPD (170 µM final) immediately followed by 10 µL of 10 mM arachidonic acid (100 µM final).

5. Using a visible spectrophotometer, either read initial rate for 10 seconds at 611 nm or take an endpoint reading at 1 minute.

6. Subtract blank from sample and calculate rate of reaction as change in optical density (OD) units.

## Observation

| S. no. | Optical density (OD) units | | |
| | Control | Test | Standard |
| --- | --- | --- | --- |
| 1. | | | |
| 2. | | | |
| 3. | | | |

**Calculation:** Rate of reaction as change in OD units per minute using the following equation:

(OD units/min) (mM TMPD/13.5 OD units) (1 mol arachidonic acid/2 mol TMPD) (2 mol $O_2$/1 mol arachidonic acid) (liter/x mg enzyme) = mmol $O_2$/min-mg.

*Note:* The extinction coefficient assumes a path length of 1 cm.

## Bibliography

1. Orlando, BJ, and Malkowski, MG (2016). Substrate-selective inhibition of cyclooxygeanse-2 by fenamic acid derivatives is dependent on peroxide tone. Journal of Biological Chemistry, 291(29), 15069–15081.

2. Vasiljevic, D, Veselinovic, M, Jovanovic, M, Jeremic, N, Arsic, A, Vucic, V, and Jakovljevic, V (2016). Evaluation of the effects of different supplementation on oxidative status in patients with rheumatoid arthritis. Clinical Rheumatology, 35(8), 1909–1915.

**EXPERIMENT 2.9**

**Aim:** To study the *in vitro* COX inhibition potential of the given sample by using prostaglandin E2 enzyme-linked immunosorbent assay (PGE2 ELISA).

**Principle:** The COX activity in cells and crude enzyme preparations may be determined by measuring prostaglandin produced on exposure to arachidonic acid. The ability to measure prostaglandins by ELISA allows for high-throughput evaluation of samples. The assays described in this protocol are for a 96-well microtiter plate format. The method provides a means for studying the inhibition of PGE2 production by small molecules, thus providing structure-activity information important for designing new molecules. In addition, the PGE2 ELISA can be used to measure endogenous prostaglandins in tissue.

## Requirements

*Chemicals*: Affinity-purified goat antirabbit immunoglobulin G (IgG); Jackson Immuno research, 50 mM potassium phosphate, pH 7.4, saturation buffer, insect cells expressing COX-1 or COX-2, cell harvest buffer, 10% (w/v) 3-[(3-cholamidopropyl)dimethylammonio]-1-propanesulfonate (CHAPS) inhibitors, including standard inhibitor (e.g. indomethacin or diclofenac), dimethylsulfoxide (DMSO) 10 mM arachidonic acid, diluted to 100 µM, prostaglandin E2 (PGE2) assay buffer with and without 20 µM indomethacin, wash buffer, prostaglandin E2 standard, ELISA buffer, PGE2-acetylcholinesterase tracer, anti-PGE2 monoclonal antibody (Cayman), and Ellman's solution.

*Equipment*: 96-well NUNC-immuno plate, MaxiSorp type 96-well round-bottom plate multichannel pipet (0–50 µL and 50–300 µL sizes) 96-well plate sealer, plate washer 96-well microplate reader.

*Glasswares*: Beakers, pipettes, measuring cylinder and glass rod.

## Procedure

**Prepare plates for ELISA** (block nonspecific interactions with reaction vessel)

1. Coat wells of a 96-well NUNC-immuno plate with the secondary antibody, affinity purified antirabbit IgG, at 8 µg/well in 200 µL of 50 mM potassium phosphate, pH 7.4, and let stand overnight at room temperature.

2. The next day, remove secondary antibody. For kinetic analysis, add the enzyme last, in which case the enzyme should be reconstituted with heme

before use (1 M heme, 5 minutes). The amount of enzyme can be varied depending on purity. Reactions can be performed at room temperature. Antibody solution and block uncoated sites on the plates by adding 100 µL saturation buffer and incubate for 6 hours. Store plates up to several months at 4°C wrapped in plastic wrap.

**Prepare enzyme**

3. Suspend intact insect cells expressing COX-1 or COX-2 1:10 (w/v) in cell harvest buffer. Centrifuge 20 min at 10,000 × g at 4°C, and suspend cells in the same buffer.

4. Add 10% CHAPS to 1% (w/v) and stir for 30 minutes using a magnetic stirrer. Pellet cell debris by centrifuging 30 minutes at 50,000 × g at 4°C. Decant and save the supernatant by freezing at −80°C. Thaw aliquots before use and keep on ice during use. Protein content is measured by the Bradford assay with BSA.

**Prepare inhibitors**

5. Dissolve inhibitors in an appropriate solvent (e.g. DMSO) as stock 10 mM solutions. Prepare duplicate or triplicate serial dilutions at 20 × final reaction concentration in a master 96-well round-bottom plate using a multichannel pipet and the solvent. Cover with a 96-well plate sealer until needed. The master plate is needed to prepare assay plates in step 6. Initially, perform the assay using seven dilutions of inhibitor ranging from 1 mM to 1 nM final.

6. Transfer 10 µL aliquots of the inhibitor dilutions from the master plate to a 96-well round-bottom assay plate.

7. For control assays, place the solvent used to dissolve inhibitors in the control wells on every plate along with serial dilutions of a standard inhibitor.

**Perform enzyme assay**

8. Add 170 µL enzyme preparation from step 3 (diluted 50- to 300-fold) with a multichannel pipet to the plate containing the inhibitors. Incubate inhibitors with enzyme for 10 minutes at 25°C. Perform reactions in duplicate or triplicate.

9. To minimize aging of the enzyme, the plate of inhibitors may be prepared prior to enzyme preparation. This assay may also be performed with purified enzyme (purified COX-1 and COX-2 are available from Cayman). Store the enzyme preparation in 1 mL aliquots at −80°C and thaw just prior to use. For the enzyme assay, dilute the enzyme stock with PGE2 assay buffer to give 0.1–1 g purified protein per 200 L reaction.

10. Initiate the reaction by adding 20 µL of 100 µM arachidonic acid (10 µM final). Mix the reaction mixture with a multichannel pipet. Let reaction proceed for 10 minutes at 25°C.

11. Terminate the reaction by transferring an aliquot of the reaction mixture to a microtiter plate with PGE2 assay buffer containing 25 µM indomethacin. The reaction mixture/PGE2 assay buffer/indomethacin solution is the source of test samples in the ELISA (step 14). The size of the aliquot depends on enzyme activity and ELISA sensitivity. Measure PGE2 by ELISA.

12. Wash plate containing secondary antibody (prepared in step 1) 3 times with wash buffer, using a plate washer.

13. To construct the standard curve, add a series of concentrations of PGE2 standard to wells on each plate (50 µL of each concentration). The concentration of PGE2 standard depends on the antibody titer, but a range of 0.04–20 ng/mL is recommended.

14. For test samples, add sample and ELISA buffer to sample wells such that µL sample + µL buffer = 50 µL.

15. Prepare PGE2-acetylcholinesterase tracer according to manufacturer's instructions. Add 50 µL tracer to each well. Store unused tracer up to 4 weeks at 4°C. Maximal response of the PGE2 assay is determined for each lot of PGE2-acetylcholinesterase by incubation with serial dilutions of antibody, prior to use in this ELISA.

16. Add 50 µL of appropriate dilution of anti-PGE2 antibody to all wells except the blank. Cover plate with a plate sealer and incubate overnight at room temperature. Either polyclonal or monoclonal antibodies may be used in this assay. The assay is based on competition between unlabeled and (enzyme) labeled prostaglandin for a limited number of specific antibody binding sites. Empirically determine the dilution of antibody giving the maximal response with the trace prior to use in this ELISA.

17. After incubation, wash plate 3 times with wash buffer. Add 200 µL Ellman's solution per well. Cover plate with a plate sealer and incubate at 37°C until control wells reach an OD412 of 1.0–1.2 (as determined using a 96-well microplate reader). If possible, place plates on a shaker where the plates can be protected from light.

18. Record data with the aid of plate reader software and calculate PGE2 levels from the standard curve determined on each plate.

## Bibliography

1. Goren, I, Lee, SY, Maucher, D, Nüsing, R, Schlich, T, Pfeilschifter, J, and Frank, S (2017). Inhibition of cyclooxygenase-1 and -2 activity in keratinocytes inhibits PGE2 formation and impairs vascular endothelial growth factor release and neovascularisation in skin wounds. International Wound Journal, 14(1), 53–63.

2. Yang, EJ, Hyun, KH, Kim, H, Kim, MJ, Lee, NH, and Hyun, CG (2016). Acanthopanax koreanum roots inhibit the expression of pro-inflammatory cytokines, inducible nitric oxide synthase, and cyclooxygenase-2 in RAW 264.7 macrophages. Oriental Journal of Chemistry, 32(1), 29–35.

# CHAPTER 3

# *In vitro* Antioxidant Assay

Oxidative stress has traditionally been viewed as a stochastic process of cell damage, wherein the process of oxidation in the human body damages cell membranes and other structures including cellular proteins, lipids and DNA.

**Etiology:** Oxidation can be accelerated by stress, cigarette smoking, alcohol, sunlight, pollution and other factors.

**Symptoms:** Some of the degenerative conditions caused by free radicals include:
- Deterioration of the eye lens, which contributes to blindness.
- Inflammation of the joints (arthritis).
- Damage to nerve cells in the brain, which contributes to conditions such as Parkinson's or Alzheimer's disease.
- Acceleration of the aging process.
- Increased risk of coronary heart disease, since free radicals encourage low-density lipoprotein (LDL) cholesterol to adhere to artery walls.
- Certain cancers, triggered by damaged cell DNA.

**Pathophysiology:** When oxygen is metabolised, it creates 'free radicals' which steal electrons from other molecules, causing damage. The body can cope with some free radicals and needs them to function effectively. However, an overload of free radicals has been linked to certain diseases, including heart disease, liver disease and some cancers.

## Bibliography

1. Dalle-Donne, I, Rossi, R, Colombo, R, Giustarini, D, and Milzani, A (2006). Biomarkers of oxidative damage in human disease. Clinical Chemistry, 52(4), 601–623.
2. Poprac, P, Jomova, K, Simunkova, M, Kollar, V, Rhodes, CJ, and Valko, M (2017). Targeting Free Radicals in Oxidative Stress-Related Human Diseases. Trends in Pharmacological Sciences, 592–607.

## EXPERIMENT 3.1

**Aim:** To study the *in vitro* antioxidant potential of the given sample by DPPH scavenging activity.

**Principle:** 1, 1-diphenyl-2-picrylhydrazyl ($\alpha,\alpha$-diphenyl-$\beta$-picrylhydrazyl) (DPPH) is a dark-colored crystalline powder composed of stable free-radical molecules. DPPH in laboratory research is used to monitor chemical reactions involving radicals, most notably it is a common antioxidant assay. It is characterized as a stable free radical by virtue of the delocalisation of the spare electron over the molecule as a whole, so that the molecule does not dimerize, as would be the case with most other free radicals. The delocalization of electron also gives rise to the deep violet color, characterized by an absorption band in ethanol solution centered at about 517 nm. When a solution of DPPH is mixed with that of a substrate (AH) that can donate a hydrogen atom, it gives rise to the reduced form with the loss of this violet color. In order to evaluate the antioxidant potential through free radical scavenging by the test samples, the change in absorbance of DPPH radicals is monitored.

### Requirements

*Chemicals:* Ascorbic acid or butylated hydroxy anisole (BHA), test sample, ethanol, Tris HCl buffer (pH 7.4), DPPH.

*Equipment:* UV-visible spectrophotometer.

*Glasswares:* Test tubes, pipettes, measuring cylinder and glass rod.

### Procedure

1. In a test tube take 0.2 mL of ethanolic solution of sample extract and add 0.8 mL of tris HCl buffer (100 mM, pH 7.4) to it.
2. To the above mentioned reaction mixture, add 1 mL of DPPH solution (500 mM in 1.0 mL ethanol).
3. Vigorously shake the mixture and incubated the same at room temperature for 30 minutes.
4. After 30 minutes, measure absorbance at 517 nm by using a UV-visible spectrophotometer.
5. Take ethanolic solution of sample extract as black and DPPH ethanolic solution as control.
6. BHA or ascorbic acid will serve as reference standard.

7. Perform the experiment in triplicates.
8. Record absorbance and calculate antioxidant potential of both test and standard according to the prescribed formula.

## Observation

| S. no. | Absorbance of control | Absorbance of test | Absorbance of standard |
|--------|----------------------|--------------------|------------------------|
| 1. | | | |
| 2. | | | |
| 3. | | | |

**Calculation:** The percentage DPPH radical scavenging activity is calculated as follows:

$$\% \text{ DPPH radical scavenging activity} = \frac{(\text{Abs control} - \text{Abs sample})}{\text{Abs control}} \times 100$$

where,   Abs control—absorbance of control

Abs sample—absorbance of sample

## Bibliography

1. Sharma, US, and Kumar, A (2011). *In vitro* antioxidant activity of Rubus ellipticus fruits. Journal of Advanced Pharmaceutical Technology and Research, 2(1), 47–50.
2. Shi, MJ, Wei, X, Xu, J, Chen, BJ, Zhao, DY, Cui, S, and Zhou, T (2017). Carboxymethylated degraded polysaccharides from Enteromorpha prolifera: Preparation and *in vitro* antioxidant activity. Food Chemistry, 215, 76–83.

## EXPERIMENT 3.2

**Aim:** To study the *in vitro* anti-inflammatory potential of the given sample by hydrogen peroxide scavenging ($H_2O_2$) assay.

**Principle:** Human beings are exposed to $H_2O_2$ indirectly via the environment nearly about 0.28 mg/kg/day with intake mostly from leaf crops. Hydrogen peroxide may enter into the human body through inhalation of vapor or mist and through eye or skin contact. $H_2O_2$ is rapidly decomposed into oxygen and water and this may produce hydroxyl radicals (OH) that can initiate lipid peroxidation and cause DNA damage in the body.

### Requirements

*Chemicals:* Ascorbic acid or butylated hydroxy anisole (BHA), test sample, phosphate buffer (pH 7.4), hydrogen peroxide, dimethyl sulfoxide (DMSO) and distill water.

*Equipment:* UV-visible spectrophotometer.

*Glasswares:* Test tubes, pipettes, measuring cylinder and glass rod.

### Procedure

1. Prepare 20 mM hydrogen peroxide solution in phosphate buffer (pH 7.4).
2. In a test tube take 2 mL of the hydrogen peroxide solution in phosphate buffer saline pH 7.4 and add 1 mL of the test sample solution prepared in distilled water.

   (Nonpolar samples that are insoluble in water are first suspended in DMSO then their aqueous solutions are prepared in distill water.)
3. Vigorously shake the mixture and incubated the same at room temperature for 10 minutes.
4. After 10 minutes, measure absorbance at 230 nm by using a UV-visible spectrophotometer against a blank solution containing the phosphate buffer without hydrogen peroxide.
5. Take hydrogen peroxide solution prepared in phosphate buffer as control and BHA or ascorbic acid will serve as reference standard.
6. Perform the experiment in triplicates.
7. Record absorbance and calculate antioxidant potential of both test and standard according to the prescribed formula.

## Observation

| S. no. | Absorbance of control | Absorbance of test | Absorbance of standard |
|--------|----------------------|--------------------|------------------------|
| 1. | | | |
| 2. | | | |
| 3. | | | |

**Calculation:** The percentage $H_2O_2$ scavenging activity is calculated as follows:

$$\% \ H_2O_2 \text{ scavenging activity} = \frac{(\text{Abs control} - \text{Abs sample})}{\text{Abs control}} \times 100$$

where, Abs control—absorbance of control

Abs sample—absorbance of sample

## Alternate Method

1. The $H_2O_2$ scavenging capacity can also be measured by dissolving 1.0 mL of 0.1 mM $H_2O_2$ (freshly made), 1.0 mL of sample solution, 0.10 mL of ammonium molybdate (3%, w/w), 10 mL of 2 M $H_2SO_4$, and 7 mL of 1.8 M KI.

2. Titrate the mixture against 5 mM $Na_2S_2O_3$ until the color disappeared. L-ascorbic acid (1000 mg/mL) is used as the positive control. The scavenging activity is calculated as:

$$\% \ H_2O_2 \text{ scavenging activity} = \frac{(V_0 - V_1)}{V_0} \times 100$$

where $V_0$—volume of $Na_2S_2O_3$ solution used to titrate the control mixture

$V_1$—volume titrated of the mixture containing the samples

## Bibliography

1. Brizzolari, A, Campisi, GM, Santaniello, E, Razzaghi-Asl, N, Saso, L, and Foti, MC (2017). Effect of organic co-solvents in the evaluation of the hydroxyl radical scavenging activity by the 2-deoxyribose degradation assay: The paradigmatic case of α-lipoic acid. Biophysical Chemistry, 220, 1–6.

2. Kerche-Silva, LE, Cavalcante, DGSM, Danna, CS, Gomes, AS, Carrara, IM, Cecchini, AL, and Job, AE (2017). Free-radical Scavenging properties and Cytotoxic Activity Evaluation of Latex C-serum from Hevea brasiliensis RRIM 600. Free Radicals and Antioxidants, 7(1), 107.

3. Olivier, MT, Muganza, FM, Shai, LJ, Gololo, SS, and Nemutavhanani, LD (2017). Phytochemical screening, antioxidant and antibacterial activities of ethanol extracts of Asparagus suaveolens aerial parts. South African Journal of Botany, 108, 41–46.

## EXPERIMENT 3.3

**Aim:** To study the *in vitro* antioxidant potential of the given sample by nitric oxide scavenging activity.

**Principle:** Nitric oxide radical is generated in biological tissues by specific nitric oxide synthases, which metabolizes arginine to citrulline with the formation of NO radical via oxidative reaction. The compound sodium nitroprusside is known to decompose in aqueous solution at physiological pH (7.2) producing nitric oxide radical. Under aerobic conditions, nitric oxide radical reacts with oxygen to produce stable products (nitrate and nitrite), the quantities of which can be determined using Griess reagent.

### Requirements

*Chemicals:* Ascorbic acid or butylated hydroxy anisole (BHA), test sample, sodium nitroprusside, phosphate buffer and griesse reagent (1:1 mixture of 0.1% naphthylethylenediamine HCl in distilled $H_2O$ and 1% sulfanilamide in 5% $H_3PO_4$).

*Equipment:* UV-visible spectrophotometer and incubator.

*Glasswares:* Test tubes, pipettes, measuring cylinder and glass rod.

### Procedure

1. In a test tube mix 0.5 mL of sample solution with 2 mL of 10 mM sodium nitroprusside dissolved in 0.5 mL of phosphate buffer saline.
2. Incubated the reaction mixture at 25°C for 150 minutes. After incubation pipette out 0.5 mL of the reaction mixture and mix with equal volume of Griess reagent.
3. Again incubate at room temperature for 30 minutes and measure absorbance at 546 nm using a UV-visible spectrophotometer against a blank solution containing the phosphate buffer without sodium nitroprusside.
4. Take sodium nitroprusside solution prepared in phosphate buffer as control and BHA or ascorbic acid will serve as reference standard.
5. Perform the experiment in triplicates.
6. Record the absorbances and calculate antioxidant potential of both test and standard according to the prescribed formula.

## Observation

| S. no. | Absorbance of control | Absorbance of test | Absorbance of standard |
|--------|----------------------|--------------------|-----------------------|
| 1. | | | |
| 2. | | | |
| 3. | | | |

**Calculation:** The percentage NO scavenging activity is calculated as follows:

$$\% \text{ NO scavenging activity} = \frac{(\text{Abs control} - \text{Abs sample})}{\text{Abs control}} \times 100$$

where, Abs control—absorbance of control

Abs sample—absorbance of sample

## Bibliography

1. Kerche-Silva, LE, Cavalcante, DGSM, Danna, CS, Gomes, AS, Carrara, IM, Cecchini, AL, and Job, AE (2017). Free-radical Scavenging properties and Cytotoxic Activity Evaluation of Latex C-serum from Hevea brasiliensis RRIM 600. Free Radicals and Antioxidants, 7(1), 107.

2. Lu, Y, Wang, A, Shi, P, and Zhang, H. (2017). A Theoretical Study on the Antioxidant Activity of Piceatannol and Isorhapontigenin Scavenging Nitric Oxide and Nitrogen Dioxide Radicals. PloS One, 12(1), e0169773.

## EXPERIMENT 3.4

**Aim:** To study the *in vitro* antioxidant potential of the given sample by reducing power method.

**Principle:** This method is based on the principle of increase in the absorbance of the reaction mixtures. Increase in the absorbance indicates an increase in the antioxidant activity. In this method, antioxidant compound forms a colored complex with potassium ferricyanide, trichloro acetic acid and ferric chloride, which is measured at 700 nm. Increase in absorbance of the reaction mixture indicates the reducing power of the samples.

### Requirements

*Chemicals:* Ascorbic acid or butylated hydroxy anisole (BHA), test sample, potassium ferricyanide [$K_3Fe(CN)_6$] , phosphate buffer (pH 6.6) trichloroacetic acid and ferric chloride [$FeCl_3$].

*Equipment:* UV-visible spectrophotometer and incubator.

*Glasswares:* Test tubes, pipettes, measuring cylinder and glass rod.

### Procedure

1. In a test tube add 2.5 mL of 0.2 M phosphate buffer (pH 6.6) and 2.5 mL of $K_3Fe(CN)_6$ (1% w/v) are added to 1.0 mL of sample dissolved in distilled water.
2. Incubate the resulting mixture at 50°C for 20 minutes, followed by the addition of 2.5 mL of trichloroaceticacid (10% w/v).
3. Centrifuge the mixture at 3000 rpm for 10 minutes to collect the upper layer of the solution (2.5 mL), mix it with distilled water (2.5 mL) and 0.5 mL of $FeCl_3$ (0.1%, w/v).
4. Measure absorbance at 700 nm using a UV-visible spectrophotometer against a blank solution containing the phosphate buffer without potassium ferricyanide.
5. Take potassium ferricyanide solution prepared in phosphate buffer as control and BHA or ascorbic acid will serve as reference standard.
6. Perform the experiment in triplicates.
7. Record the absorbances and calculate antioxidant potential of both test and standard according to the prescribed formula.

## Observation

| S. no. | Absorbance of control | Absorbance of test | Absorbance of standard |
|---|---|---|---|
| 1. | | | |
| 2. | | | |
| 3. | | | |

**Calculation:** The percentage reducing power is calculated as follows:

$$\% \text{ reducing power} = \frac{(\text{Abs control} - \text{Abs sample})}{\text{Abs control}} \times 100$$

where,  Abs control—absorbance of control

Abs sample—absorbance of sample

## Bibliography

1. Jena, S, Ray, A, Banerjee, A, Sahoo, A, Nasim, N, Sahoo, S, and Nayak, S (2017). Chemical composition and antioxidant activity of essential oil from leaves and rhizomes of Curcuma angustifolia Roxb. Natural Product Research, 1–4.

2. Olivier, MT, Muganza, FM, Shai, LJ, Gololo, SS, and Nemutavhanani, LD (2017). Phytochemical screening, antioxidant and antibacterial activities of ethanol extracts of Asparagus suaveolens aerial parts. South African Journal of Botany, 108, 41–46.

## EXPERIMENT 3.5

**Aim:** To study the *in vitro* antioxidant potential of the given sample by total antioxidant capacity assay (phosphomolybdenum method).

**Principle:** This method is a spectroscopic method for the quantitative determination of antioxidant capacity, through the formation of phosphomolybdenum complex. The assay is based on the reduction of Mo(VI) to Mo(V) by the sample analyte and subsequent formation of a green phosphate Mo(V) complex at acidic pH.

### Requirements

*Chemicals:* Ascorbic acid or butylated hydroxy anisole (BHA), test sample, sulfuric acid, sodium phosphate and ammonium molybdate.

*Equipment:* UV-visible spectrophotometer and water bath.

*Glasswares:* Test tubes, pipettes, measuring cylinder and glass rod.

### Procedure

1. In a test tube add 0.1 mL of sample (100 µg) solution combined with 1 mL of reagent (0.6 M sulfuric acid, 28 mM sodium phosphate and 4 mM ammonium molybdate).
2. Cap the test tube and incubated in a boiling water bath at 95°C for 90 minutes.
3. After cooling the sample to room temperature, measure absorbance of the aqueous solution at 695 nm against blank in UV spectrophotometer. A typical blank solution contained 1 mL of reagent solution and the appropriate volume of the same solvent used for the sample and it is incubated under same conditions as rest of the sample.
4. Take BHA or ascorbic acid will serve as reference standard.
5. Perform the experiment in triplicates.
6. Record the absorbances and calculate total antioxidant capacity of both test and standard according to the prescribed formula.

### Observation

| S. no. | Absorbance of control | Absorbance of test | Absorbance of standard |
|--------|----------------------|--------------------|------------------------|
| 1. | | | |
| 2. | | | |
| 3. | | | |

**Calculation:** Total antioxidant capacity is calculated as follows:

$$\text{Total antioxidant capacity} = \frac{(\text{Abs control} - \text{Abs sample})}{\text{Abs control}} \times 100$$

where, Abs control—absorbance of control
Abs sample—absorbance of sample

## Bibliography

1. Kerche-Silva, LE, Cavalcante, DGSM, Danna, CS, Gomes, AS, Carrara, IM, Cecchini, AL, and Job, AE (2017). Free-radical Scavenging properties and Cytotoxic Activity Evaluation of Latex C-serum from Hevea brasiliensis RRIM 600. Free Radicals and Antioxidants, 7(1), 107.

2. Paraskeuas, V, Fegeros, K, Hunger, C, Theodorou, G, and Mountzouris, KC (2017). Dietary inclusion level effects of a phytogenic characterised by menthol and anethole on broiler growth performance, biochemical parameters including total antioxidant capacity and gene expression of immune-related biomarkers. Animal Production Science, 57(1), 33–41.

## EXPERIMENT 3.6

**Aim:** To study the *in vitro* antioxidant potential of the given sample by ferric reducing antioxidant power (FRAP) assay.

**Principle:** A simple, automated test measuring the ferric reducing ability of plasma, the FRAP assay, is presented as a viable method for assessing 'antioxidant power.' Ferric to ferrous ion reduction at low pH causes a colored ferrous-tripyridyltriazine complex to form. FRAP values are obtained by comparing the absorbance change at 593 nm in test reaction mixtures with those containing ferrous ions in known concentration.

### Requirements

*Chemicals:* Ascorbic acid or butylated hydroxy anisole (BHA), test sample, acetate buffer (pH 3.6), 2,4,6-tripyridyl-s-triazine (TPTZ), hydrochloric acid and ferric chloride.

*Equipment:* UV-visible spectrophotometer and water bath.

*Glasswares:* Test tubes, pipettes, measuring cylinder and glass rod.

### Procedure

1. Prepare FRAP reagent by dissolving 200 mL acetate buffer (pH 3.6), 2.5 mL of 10 mM TPTZ in 40 mM HCl, and adding 2.5 mL of 20 mM ferric chloride to the resulting solution.
2. Mix 3 mL of prepared FRAP reagent with 100 µL of diluted sample.
3. Incubate the mixture at 37°C for 30 minutes and measure absorbance at 593 nm against blank (FRAP reagent + distilled water).
4. Take BHA or ascorbic acid will serve as reference standard.
5. Perform the experiment in triplicates.
6. Record absorbance and calculate antioxidant capacity of both test and standard according to the prescribed formula.

### Observation

| S. no. | Absorbance of control | Absorbance of test | Absorbance of standard |
|--------|----------------------|--------------------|------------------------|
| 1. | | | |
| 2. | | | |
| 3. | | | |

**Calculation:** Total antioxidant capacity is calculated as follows:

$$\text{Total antioxidant capacity} = \frac{(\text{Abs control} - \text{Abs sample})}{\text{Abs control}} \times 100$$

where,   Abs control—absorbance of control

Abs sample—absorbance of sample

## Bibliography

1. Al-Rimawi, F, Abu-Lafi, S, Abbadi, J, Alamarneh, AA, Sawahreh, RA, and Odeh, I (2017). Analysis of phenolic and flavonoids of wild ephedra alata plant extracts by lc/pda and lc/ms and their antioxidant activity. African Journal of Traditional, Complementary and Alternative Medicines (AJTCAM), 14(2), 130–141.

2. Hua, R, Cheng, D, Coyaud, É, Freeman, S, Di Pietro, E, Wang, Y, and Brumell, JH (2017). VAPs and ACBD5 tether peroxisomes to the ER for peroxisome maintenance and lipid homeostasis. J Cell Biol, JCB-201608128.

## EXPERIMENT 3.7

**Aim:** To study the *in vitro* antioxidant potential of the given sample by xanthine oxidase activity.

**Principle:** Uric acid is a breakdown product of ingested and endogenously synthesized purines. DNA and RNA are degraded into purine nucleotides and bases, which are then metabolized, via the action of xanthine oxidase, to xanthine and uric acid. Xanthine oxidase (XO) belongs to the molybdenum-protein family and functions to catalyse the oxidation of hypoxanthine to xanthine and subsequently to uric acid. During the reoxidation of XO, molecular oxygen acts as electron acceptor, producing reactive oxygen species (ROS) such as hydrogen peroxide, superoxide radical anion, hydroxyl radical, alkylperoxyl radical, nitric oxide, and singlet oxygen that are often associated with a wide variety of degenerative processes and diseases. Thus, overactivity of XO results in a condition known as gout, a common rheumatic disease and an acute inflammatory arthritis and also certain vascular degenerative diseases. The inhibition of XO reduces both vascular oxidative stress and circulating levels of uric acid. The following method of testing antioxidant potential of the test sample is based on determining spectrophotometrically the inhibitory potential of sample on the xanthine oxidase activity with xanthine as sub-substrate.

### Requirements

*Chemicals:* Ascorbic acid or butylated hydroxy anisole (BHA), test sample, phosphate buffer (pH 7.5), xanthine oxidase, xanthine substrate solution and hydrochloric acid and allopurinol.

*Equipment:* UV-visible spectrophotometer and water bath.

*Glasswares:* Test tubes, pipettes, measuring cylinder and glass rod.

### Procedure

1. In a test tube mix sample drug or extract (500 µL of 0.1 mg/mL) and allopurinol (100 µg/mL) (in methanol) with 1.3 mL phosphate buffer (0.05 M, pH 7.5) and 0.2 mL of 0.2 units/mL xanthine oxidase solution.

2. Incubate the mixture at room temperature for 10 minutes and add 1.5 mL of 0.15 M xanthine substrate solution to this mixture.

3. Again incubate the mixture for 30 minutes at room temperature (25°C) and then measure absorbance at 293 nm using a spectrophotometer against blank (0.5 mL methanol, 1.3 mL phosphate buffer, and 0.2 mL xanthine oxidase).

4. Use solution of 0.5 mL methanol, 1.3 mL phosphate buffer, 0.2 mL xanthine oxidase and 1.5 mL xanthine substrate as control.
5. Take BHA or ascorbic acid will serve as reference standard.
6. Perform the experiment in triplicates.
7. Record absorbance and calculate percentage inhibition of xanthine oxidase activity of both test and standard according to the prescribed formula.

## Observation

| S. no. | Absorbance of control | Absorbance of test | Absorbance of standard |
|--------|----------------------|--------------------|------------------------|
| 1. | | | |
| 2. | | | |
| 3. | | | |

**Calculation:** Percentage inhibition of xanthine oxidase activity is calculated as follows:

$$\% \text{ inhibition} = \frac{(\text{Abs control} - \text{Abs sample})}{\text{Abs control}} \times 100$$

where, Abs control—absorbance of control

Abs sample—absorbance of sample

## Bibliography

1. Kostić, DA, Dimitrijević, DS, Stojanović, GS, Palić, IR, Đordević, AS, and Ickovski, JD (2015). Xanthine oxidase: isolation, assays of activity, and inhibition. Journal of Chemistry, 2015.
2. Lin, KW, Chen, YT, Yang, SC, Wei, BL, Hung, CF, and Lin, CN (2013). Xanthine oxidase inhibitory lanostanoids from Ganoderma tsugae. Fitoterapia, 89, 231–238.

## EXPERIMENT 3.8

**Aim:** To study the *in vitro* antioxidant potential of the given sample by hydroxyl (HO˙) radical scavenging assay.

**Principle:** It is commonly believed that the *in vivo* damage of biomolecules is initiated by reactive oxygen species (ROS) in a process known as oxidative stress. In living organisms there are two major reactive oxygen species, superoxide radical and hydroxyl radical that are being continuously formed in a process of reduction of oxygen to water. Hydroxyl radical is one of the potent reactive oxygen species in the biological system that reacts with polyunsaturated fatty acid moieties of cell membrane phospholipids and causes damage to cell. HO˙ radicals were generated from $FeSO_4$ and $H_2O_2$, and detected by their ability to hydroxylate salicylate.

## Requirements

*Chemicals:* Ascorbic acid or butylated hydroxy anisole (BHA), test sample, ferric sulphate, hydrogen peroxide and sodium salicylate.
*Equipment:* UV-visible spectrophotometer and water bath.
*Glasswares:* Test tubes, pipettes, measuring cylinder and glass rod.

## Procedure

1. In a test tube mix reaction mixture (2 mL) containing 0.5 mL $FeSO_4$ (1.5 mM), 0.35 mL $H_2O_2$ (6 mM), 0.15 mL sodium salicylate (20 mM), and 1 mL of sample solution.
2. Incubate the mixture at 37°C for 60 minutes and add 1.5 mL of 0.15 M xanthine substrate solution is to this mixture.
3. Measure absorbance at 562 nm using a spectrophotometer against blank.
4. Take BHA or ascorbic acid will serve as reference standard.
5. Perform the experiment in triplicates.
6. Record absorbance and calculate percentage hydroxyl radical scavenging activity of both test and standard according to the prescribed formula.

## Observation

| S. no. | Absorbance of control | Absorbance of test | Absorbance of standard |
|--------|----------------------|--------------------|------------------------|
| 1. | | | |
| 2. | | | |
| 3. | | | |

**Calculation:** Hydroxyl radical scavenging activity is calculated as follows:

$$\text{Hydroxyl radical scavenging activity} = \frac{(\text{Abs control} - \text{Abs sample})}{\text{Abs control}} \times 100$$

where,  Abs control—absorbance of control
Abs sample—absorbance of sample

## Bibliography

1. Kerche-Silva, LE, Cavalcante, DGSM, Danna, CS, Gomes, AS, Carrara, IM, Cecchini, AL, and Job, AE (2017). Free-radical Scavenging properties and Cytotoxic Activity Evaluation of Latex C-serum from Hevea brasiliensis RRIM 600. Free Radicals and Antioxidants, 7(1), 107.

2. Zhang, J, Hou, X, Ahmad, H, Zhang, H, Zhang, L, and Wang, T (2014). Assessment of free radicals scavenging activity of seven natural pigments and protective effects in AAPH-challenged chicken erythrocytes. Food Chemistry, 145, 57–65.

**EXPERIMENT 3.9**

**Aim:** To study the *in vitro* antioxidant potential of the given sample by superoxide radical scavenging assay.

**Principle:** It is commonly believed that the in vivo damage of biomolecules is initiated by reactive oxygen species (ROS) in a process known as oxidative stress. In living organisms there are two major reactive oxygen species, superoxide radical and hydroxyl radical, that are being continuously formed in a process of reduction of oxygen to water. Although superoxide anion is a weak oxidant, it ultimately produces powerful and dangerous hydroxyl radicals as well as singlet oxygen, both of which contribute to oxidative stress.

## Requirements

*Chemicals:* Ascorbic acid or butylated hydroxy anisole (BHA), test sample, Tris-HCl buffer, nitroblue tetrazolium (NBT), NADH solution and phenazine methosulfate solution (PMS).

*Equipment:* UV-visible spectrophotometer and water bath.

*Glasswares:* Test tubes, pipettes, measuring cylinder and glass rod.

## Procedure

1. In a test tube generate superoxide anion radicals by dissolving 3.0 mL of Tris-HCl buffer (16 mM, pH 8.0), containing 0.5 mL of nitroblue tetrazolium (NBT) (0.3 mM), 0.5 mL NADH (0.936 mM) solution, 1.0 mL sample and 0.5 mL Tris-HCl buffer (16 mM, pH 8.0). The reaction is initiated by adding 0.5 mL phenazine methosulfate (PMS) solution (0.12 mM) to the mixture.
2. Incubate the mixture at 25 °C for 5 minutes.
3. Measure absorbance at 56 nm using a spectrophotometer against blank.
4. Take BHA or ascorbic acid will serve as reference standard.
5. Perform the experiment in triplicates.
6. Record absorbance and calculate percentage superoxide radical scavenging activity of both test and standard according to the prescribed formula.

## Observation

| S. no. | Absorbance of control | Absorbance of test | Absorbance of standard |
|--------|----------------------|--------------------|------------------------|
| 1.     |                      |                    |                        |
| 2.     |                      |                    |                        |
| 3.     |                      |                    |                        |

**Calculation:** Superoxide radical scavenging activity is calculated as follows:

$$\text{Superoxide radical scavenging activity} = \frac{(\text{Abs control} - \text{Abs sample})}{\text{Abs control}} \times 100$$

where,  Abs control—absorbance of control

Abs sample—absorbance of sample

## Bibliography

1. Kaur, G, Gupta, V, and Bansal, P (2017). Innate antioxidant activity of some traditional formulations. Journal of Advanced Pharmaceutical Technology and Research, 8(1), 39.
2. Kerche-Silva, LE, Cavalcante, DGSM, Danna, CS, Gomes, AS, Carrara, IM, Cecchini, AL, and Job, AE (2017). Free-radical Scavenging properties and Cytotoxic Activity Evaluation of Latex C-serum from Hevea brasiliensis RRIM 600. Free Radicals and Antioxidants, 7(1), 107.

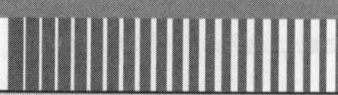

# CHAPTER 4

# *In vitro* Antidiabetic Assay

Diabetes mellitus (DM), commonly referred to as diabetes, is a group of metabolic diseases in which there are high blood sugar levels over a prolonged period.

**Types:** There are three main types of diabetes mellitus:

- Type 1 DM results from the pancreas' failure to produce enough insulin. This form was previously referred to as 'insulin-dependent diabetes mellitus' (IDDM) or 'juvenile diabetes'. The cause is unknown.

- Type 2 DM begins with insulin resistance, a condition in which cells fail to respond to insulin properly. As the disease progresses a lack of insulin may also develop. This form was previously referred to as 'noninsulin-dependent diabetes mellitus' (NIDDM) or 'adult-onset diabetes'. The most common cause is excessive body weight and not enough exercise.

- Gestational diabetes is the third main form and occurs when pregnant women without a previous history of diabetes develop high blood-sugar levels.

| Table 4.1: Blood sugar levels in diagnosing diabetes | | | |
|---|---|---|---|
| *Plasma glucose test* | *Normal* | *Prediabetes* | *Diabetes* |
| **Random** | Below 11.1 mmol/L Below 200 mg/dL | N/A | 11.1 mmol/L or more 200 mg/dL or more |
| **Fasting** | Below 6.1 mmol/L Below 108 mg/dL | 6.1–6.9 mmol/L 108–125 mg/dL | 7.0 mmol/L or more 126 mg/dL or more |
| **2 hours post-prandial** | Below 7.8 mmol/L Below 140 mg/dL | 7.8–11.0 mmol/L 140–199 mg/dL | 11.1 mmol/L or more 200 mg/dL or more |

**Symptoms:** The classic symptoms of untreated diabetes are weight loss, polyuria (increased urination), polydipsia (increased thirst), and polyphagia (increased hunger). Symptoms may develop rapidly (weeks or months) in type 1 DM, while they usually develop much more slowly and may be subtle or absent in type 2 DM. Several other signs and symptoms can mark the onset of diabetes although they are not specific to the disease. In addition to the known ones above, they include blurry vision, headache, fatigue, slow healing of cuts, and itchy skin. Prolonged high blood glucose can cause glucose absorption in the lens of the eye, which leads to changes in its shape, resulting in vision changes. A number of skin rashes that can occur in diabetes are collectively known as diabetic dermadromes.

**Diagnosis:**

- *Random plasma glucose test*: A blood sample for a random plasma glucose test can be taken at any time. This doesn't require as much planning and is therefore used in the diagnosis of type 1 diabetes when time is of the essence.

- *Fasting plasma glucose test*: A fasting plasma glucose test is taken after at least 8 hours of fasting and is therefore usually taken in the morning.

  The National Institute for Health and Care Excellence, UK (NICE) guidelines regard a fasting plasma glucose result of 5.5 mmol/L as putting someone at higher risk of developing type 2 diabetes, particularly when accompanied by other risk factors for type 2 diabetes.

- *Oral glucose tolerance test (OGTT)*: A test to determine the body's ability to handle glucose. In the test, a person fasts overnight (at least 8 hours but not more than 16 hours). Then first, the fasting plasma glucose is tested. It is currently the gold standard for the diagnosis of diabetes.

- *HbA1c test for diabetes diagnosis*: A hemoglobin 1Ac (HbA1c) test does not directly measure the level of blood glucose, however, the result of the test is influenced by how high or low your blood glucose levels have tended to be over a period of 2–3 months.

  Indications of diabetes or prediabetes are given under the following conditions:
  - Normal: Below 42 mmol/mol (6.0%)
  - Prediabetes: 42–47 mmol/mol (6.0–6.4%)
  - Diabetes: 48 mmol/mol (6.5% or over)

## Pathophysiology

Insulin is the principal hormone that regulates the uptake of glucose from the blood into most cells of the body, especially liver, adipose tissue and muscle, except smooth muscle, in which insulin acts via the insulin-like growth factor 1 (IGF-1). Therefore, deficiency of insulin or the insensitivity of its receptors plays a central role in all forms of diabetes mellitus.

The body obtains glucose from three main places—the intestinal absorption of food, the breakdown of glycogen, the storage form of glucose found in the liver, and gluconeogenesis, the generation of glucose from non-carbohydrate substrates in the body. Insulin plays a critical role in balancing glucose levels in the body. Insulin can inhibit the breakdown of glycogen or the process of gluconeogenesis, it can stimulate the transport of glucose into fat and muscle cells, and it can stimulate the storage of glucose in the form of glycogen.

Insulin is released into the blood by beta cells (β-cells), found in the islets of Langerhans in the pancreas, in response to rising levels of blood glucose, typically after eating. Insulin is used by about two-thirds of the body's cells to absorb glucose from the blood for use as fuel, for conversion to other needed molecules, or for storage. Lower glucose levels result in decreased insulin release from the beta cells and in the breakdown of glycogen to glucose. This process is mainly controlled by the hormone glucagon, which acts in the opposite manner to insulin.

If the amount of insulin available is insufficient, if cells respond poorly to the effects of insulin (insulin insensitivity or insulin resistance), or if the insulin itself is defective, then glucose will not be absorbed properly by the body cells that require it, and it will not be stored appropriately in the liver and muscles. The net effect is persistently high levels of blood glucose, poor protein synthesis, and other metabolic derangements, such as acidosis.

When the glucose concentration in the blood remains high over time, the kidneys will reach a threshold of reabsorption, and glucose will be excreted in the urine (glycosuria). This increases the osmotic pressure of the urine and inhibits reabsorption of water by the kidney, resulting in increased urine production (polyuria) and increased fluid loss. Lost blood volume will be replaced osmotically from water held in body cells and other body compartments, causing dehydration and increased thirst (polydipsia).

## Bibliography

1. Diabetes Control and Complications Trial Research Group (1993). The effect of intensive treatment of diabetes on the development and progression of long-term complications in insulin-dependent diabetes mellitus. N Engl J Med, 1993(329), 977–986.
2. Olokoba, AB, Obateru, OA, and Olokoba, LB (2012). Type 2 Diabetes Mellitus: A Review of Current Trends. Oman Medical Journal, 27(4), 269–273.

## EXPERIMENT 4.1

**Aim:** To study the *in vitro* antidiabetic potential of the given sample by determining its α-amylase inhibitory action using starch iodine method.

**Principle:** In humans, the digestion of starch involves several stages. Initially, partial digestion by the salivary amylase results in the degradation of polymeric substrates into shorter oligomers. Later on in the gut these are further hydrolyzed by pancreatic α-amylases into maltose, maltotriose and small malto-oligosaccharides. The digestive enzyme (α-amylase) is responsible for hydrolyzing dietary starch (maltose), which breaks down into glucose prior to absorption. Inhibition of α-amylase can lead to reduction in postprandial hyperglycemia in diabetic condition.

Alpha-amylase activity can be measured *in vitro* by hydrolysis of starch in presence of α-amylase enzyme. This process was quantified by using iodine, which gives blue colour with starch. The reduced intensity of blue color indicates the enzyme-induced hydrolysis of starch into monosaccharides. If the substance/extract possesses α-amylase inhibitory activity, the intensity of blue color will be more. In other words, the intensity of blue color in test sample is directly proportional to α-amylase inhibitory activity.

### Requirements

*Chemicals:* Acarbose (standard), test sample, phosphate buffer (pH 7.0), starch, iodine and distill water.

*Equipment:* UV-visible spectrophotometer.

*Glasswares:* Test tubes, micropipettes, measuring cylinder and glass rod.

### Procedure

1. Mix 10 μL of α-amylase solution (0.025 mg/L) with 390 μL of phosphate buffer (pH 7.0) containing different concentrations of the test sample.
2. Incubate at 37°C for 10 minutes and add 100 μL of 1% starch solution. Re-incubate the reaction mixture at 37°C for 1 hour.
3. After 1 hour, add 0.1 mL of 1% iodine solution and 5 mL distilled water.
4. Measure absorbance at 565 nm using UV-visible spectrophotometer.
5. Take reaction mixture devoid of α-amylase as black and mixture devoid of starch as control.
6. Acarbose will serve as reference standard.

7. Perform the experiment in triplicates.
8. Record absorbance and calculate enzyme inhibition potential of both test and standard according to the prescribed formula.

## Observation

| S. no. | Absorbance of control | Absorbance of test | Absorbance of standard |
|--------|----------------------|--------------------|------------------------|
| 1. | | | |
| 2. | | | |
| 3. | | | |

**Calculation:** The percentage inhibition of enzyme activity is calculated as follows:

$$\% \text{ inhibition of } \alpha\text{-amylase} = \frac{(\text{Abs control} - \text{Abs sample})}{\text{Abs control}} \times 100$$

where,  Abs control—absorbance of control
Abs sample—absorbance of sample

## Bibliography

1. Tundis, R, Loizzo, MR, and Menichini, F (2010). Natural products as α-amylase and α-glucosidase inhibitors and their hypoglycaemic potential in the treatment of diabetes: an update. Mini Reviews in Medicinal Chemistry, 10(4), 315–331.
2. Uddin, N, Hasan, MR, Hossain, MM, Sarker, A, Hasan, AN, Islam, AM, and Rana, MS (2014). In vitro α-amylase inhibitory activity and in vivo hypoglycemic effect of methanol extract of Citrus macroptera Montr. fruit. Asian Pacific Journal of Tropical Biomedicine, 4(6), 473–479.

## EXPERIMENT 4.2

**Aim:** To study the *in vitro* antidiabetic potential of the given sample by α-glucosidase inhibitory assay.

**Principle:** Alpha-glucosidase is a membrane bound enzyme located on the epithelium of the small intestine, catalyzing the cleavage of disaccharides to form glucose. Inhibitors can retard the uptake of dietary carbohydrates and suppress postprandial hyperglycemia. Therefore, inhibition of α-glucosidase could be one of the most effective approaches to control diabetes. Glucosidases are not only essential to carbohydrate digestion, but also vital for the processing of glycoprotein and glycolipids. This enzyme is a target for antiviral agents that interfere with the formation of essential glycoproteins required in viral assembly, secretion and infection. Glucosidases are also involved in a variety of metabolic disorders and carcinogenesis.

Alpha-glucosidase activity can be measured *in vitro* by determination of the reducing sugar (glucose) arising from hydrolysis of sucrose by α-glucosidase enzyme.

### Requirements

*Chemicals:* Acarbose (standard), test sample, phosphate buffer (pH 6.8), *p*-nitrophenyl α-D-glucopyranoside (pNPG), DMSO, α-glucosidase and sodium carbonate solution to stop the reaction and distilled water.

*Equipment:* 96-well plate and microplate reader.

*Glasswares:* Test tubes, micropipettes, measuring cylinder and glass rod.

### Procedure

1. Prepare 60 μL reaction mixture containing 20 μL of 100 mM phosphate buffer (pH 6.8), 20 μL of 2.5 mM *p*NPG in the buffer, and 20 μL of sample dissolved in 10% DMSO, and added to each well of a 96-well plate.
2. Add 20 μL of 10 mM phosphate buffer (pH 6.8) containing 0.2 U/mL α-glucosidase to the mixture.
3. Incubate the plate at 37°C for 15 minutes, then add 80 μL of 0.2 mM sodium carbonate solution to stop the reaction.
4. Right after that, record absorbance at 405 nm using a microplate reader.
5. Control will contain the same reaction mixture except the same volume of phosphate buffer is added instead of the sample solution. Acarbose dissolved in 10% DMSO is used as a positive control.

6. Perform the experiment in triplicates.
7. Record absorbance and calculate enzyme inhibition potential of both test and standard according to the prescribed formula.

## Observation

| S. no. | Absorbance of control | Absorbance of test | Absorbance of standard |
|--------|-----------------------|--------------------|------------------------|
| 1. | | | |
| 2. | | | |
| 3. | | | |

**Calculation:** The percentage inhibition of enzyme activity is calculated as follows:

$$\% \text{ inhibition of } \alpha\text{-glucosidase} = \frac{(\text{Abs control} - \text{Abs sample})}{\text{Abs control}} \times 100$$

where,  Abs control—absorbance of control
Abs sample—absorbance of sample

## Bibliography

1. Podsedek, A, Majewska, I, Redzynia, M, Sosnowska, D, and Koziolkiewicz, M (2014). *In vitro* inhibitory effect on digestive enzymes and antioxidant potential of commonly consumed fruits. Journal of Agricultural and Food Chemistry, 62(20), 4610–4617.
2. Tundis, R, Loizzo, MR, and Menichini, F (2010). Natural products as α-amylase and α-glucosidase inhibitors and their hypoglycaemic potential in the treatment of diabetes: an update. Mini Reviews in Medicinal Chemistry, 10(4), 315–331.

## EXPERIMENT 4.3

**Aim:** To study the *in vitro* antidiabetic potential of the given sample by glucose diffusion assay.

**Principle:** Glucose is a six-carbon sugar that is directly metabolized by cells to provide energy. The enteric cells of the small intestine absorb glucose along with other nutrients from the ingested food. As a glucose molecule is too large to pass through a cell membrane via simple diffusion, it gets transported through facilitated diffusion and two types of active transport. The rate of glucose transport across cell membrane is yet another important tool to evaluate the potency of antidiabetic drugs. This assay aids to evaluate the potential of drugs in inducing or inhibiting the entry of glucose inside the cells.

## Requirements

*Chemicals:* Acarbose (standard), test sample, sodium chloride, glucose and distill water.

*Equipment:* Spectrophotometer and orbital shaker.

*Glasswares:* Test tubes, micropipettes, measuring cylinder and glass rod.

## Procedure

1. Place sample solution along with a glucose solution (0.22 mM in 0.15 M sodium chloride) in a dialysis membrane (12000 MW).
2. Tie both ends of the dialysis membrane using thread and immersed in a beaker containing 40 mL of 0.15 M sodium chloride and 10 mL of distilled water.
3. Place the beakers on an orbital shaker and keep at room temperature.
4. Monitor the movement of glucose into the external solution every half hour spectrophotometrically at 260 nm.
5. The control contains 1 mL of 0.15 M sodium chloride, 22 mM glucose and 1 mL of distilled water.
6. Perform the experiment in triplicates.

## Observation

| S. no. | Absorbance of control | Absorbance of test | Absorbance of standard |
|--------|----------------------|--------------------|------------------------|
| 1. | | | |
| 2. | | | |
| 3. | | | |

**Calculation:** The percentage inhibition of glucose diffusion is calculated as follows:

$$\% \text{ inhibition of glucose diffusion} = \frac{(\text{Abs control} - \text{Abs sample})}{\text{Abs control}} \times 100$$

where,  Abs control—absorbance of control

Abs sample—absorbance of sample

## Bibliography

1. Balraj, S, Indumathy, R, Jayshree, N, and Abirami, MSA (2016). Evaluation of In vitro Anti-diabetic Activity of Various Root Extract of Cassia fistula L. Imperial Journal of Interdisciplinary Research, 2(6).
2. Kumar, A, and Jaiswal, M (2016). Effect of Self Nanoemulsifying Drug Delivery System (SNEDDS) on Intestinal Permeation and Anti-Diabetic Activity of Berberis aristata Extract: *In-Vitro* and *Ex-Vivo* Studies. Journal of Nanopharmaceutics and Drug Delivery, 3(1), 51–62.

**EXPERIMENT 4.4**

**Aim:** To study the *in vitro* antidiabetic potential of the given sample by protein tyrosine phosphatase inhibition assay.

**Principle:** Protein tyrosine phosphatase functions as a negative regulator of insulin and leptin signal transduction. Inhibition of protein tyrosine phosphatase has emerged as a highly validated, attractive target for treatment of not only diabetes but also obesity.

## Requirements

*Chemicals:* Acarbose (standard), test sample, *p*-nitrophenyl phosphate (*p*NPP) and ethylenediaminetetraacetic acid (EDTA), protein tyrosine phosphatase (PTP) 1B (human recombinant), and sodium hydroxide (NaOH).

*Equipment:* 96-well plate and microplate reader.

*Glasswares:* Test tubes, micropipettes, measuring cylinder and glass rod.

## Procedure

1. The inhibitory activity of the sample is evaluated using *p*NPP as substrate.
2. To each 96-well (final volume 110 μL) add 2 mM *p*NPP and PTP1B in a buffer containing 50 mM citrate (pH 6.0), 0.1 mM NaCl, 1 mM EDTA, and 1 mM dithiothreital (DTT) with or without sample.
3. Preincubate the plate at 37°C for 10 minutes, and then add 50 μL of *p*NPP in buffer.
4. Following incubation at 37°C for 30 minutes, terminate the reaction with the addition of 10 M NaOH.
5. The amount of *p*-nitrophenyl produced after enzymetic dephosphorylation is estimated by measuring the absorbance at 405 nm using microplate reader.
6. The nonenzymatic hydrolysis of 2 mM *p*NPP is corrected by measuring the increase in absorbance at 405 nm obtained in absence of PTP1B enzyme.
7. Perform the experiment in triplicates.
8. Record the absorbances and calculate antioxidant potential of both test and standard according to the prescribed formula.

## Observation

| S. no. | Absorbance of control | Absorbance of test | Absorbance of standard |
|--------|----------------------|--------------------|-----------------------|
| 1. | | | |
| 2. | | | |
| 3. | | | |

**Calculation:** The percentage inhibition of enzyme activity is calculated as follows:

$$\% \text{ inhibition of enzyme} = \frac{(\text{Abs control} - \text{Abs sample})}{\text{Abs control}} \times 100$$

where,   Abs control—absorbance of control

              Abs sample—absorbance of sample

## Bibliography

1. Campochiaro, PA, Sophie, R, Tolentino, M, Miller, DM, Browning, D, Boyer, DS, and Peters, K (2015). Treatment of diabetic macular edema with an inhibitor of vascular endothelial-protein tyrosine phosphatase that activates Tie2. Ophthalmology, 122(3), 545–554.
2. Choi, JS, Ali, MY, Jung, HA, Oh, SH, Choi, RJ, and Kim, EJ (2015). Protein tyrosine phosphatase 1B inhibitory activity of alkaloids from Rhizoma Coptidis and their molecular docking studies. Journal of Ethnopharmacology, 171, 28–36.

## EXPERIMENT 4.5

**Aim:** To study the *in vitro* antidiabetic potential of the given sample by glycation inhibition assay.

**Principle:** Glycation is the result of the covalent bonding of a sugar molecule, such as glucose or fructose, to a protein or lipid molecule, without the controlling action of an enzyme. During long standing hyperglycemic state in diabetes mellitus, glucose forms covalent adducts with the plasma proteins through a nonenzymatic process known as glycation. Protein glycation and formation of advanced glycation end products (AGEs) play an important role in the pathogenesis of diabetic complications like retinopathy, nephropathy, neuropathy, cardiomyopathy along with some other diseases such as rheumatoid arthritis, osteoporosis and aging. Glycation of proteins interferes with their normal functions by disrupting molecular conformation, altering enzymatic activity, and interfering with receptor functioning. AGEs form intra- and extracellular cross-linking not only with proteins, but also with some other endogenous key molecules including lipids and nucleic acids to contribute in the development of diabetic complications. Recent studies suggest that AGEs interact with plasma membrane localized receptors for AGEs (RAGE) to alter intracellular signaling, gene expression, release of proinflammatory molecules and free radicals.

## Requirements

*Chemicals:* Acarbose (standard), test sample, oxalic acid, TBA phosphate buffer saline (PBS), trichloroacetic acid, $NaBH_4$ and distilled water.

*Equipment:* Spectrophotometer.

*Glasswares:* Test tubes, micropipettes, measuring cylinder and glass rod.

## Procedure

1. To study the effect of sample on protein glycation process, fifteen combinations of 0.075 M phosphate buffer saline with glucose (G1: 5.5, G2: 25, G3: 50 mM), sample drug (I1:5, I2:10, I3:20, I4: 40 g/L as inhibitor) and protein (bovine albumin) is incubated at 37°C for 5 weeks.
2. Samples are analyzed after third and fifth weeks of incubation.
3. Glucose concentrations is measured and samples are dialyzed to remove free glucose. Free glucose is the major hindrance in estimation of glycation level.

4. Postdialysis, glucose was again estimated to confirm final glucose levels.

5. Total proteins after dialysis is determined by biuret method.

6. 1 mL of dialyzed sample (total protein = 10 mg/mL) is used for non-enzymatic and enzymatic glycation.

### Nonenzymatic and Enzymatic Glycation

1. Arrange three test tubes for each of the reduced and nonreduced samples. Add 0.1 mL of $NaBH_4$ in the reduced samples and 0.1 mL of 0.01 N NaOH to the nonreduced samples.

2. Leave all test tubes undisturbed for 30 minutes at 37°C. After half an hour, add 1 drop of 1N HCl in each test tube, followed by addition of 0.5 mL oxalic acid.

3. Cap the tubes and autoclave for half an hour at 124°C (115 lb/inch² pressure). Cool the tubes to room temperature and then place in ice.

4. Add in each tube, 0.5 mL of 40% trichloroacetic acid (chilled). Afterwards, centrifuge the samples for 15 minutes at 15000 rpm.

5. Mix the supernatant (1.5 mL) with 0.5 mL freshly prepared TBA. Incubate the samples at 37°C in water bath for 15 minutes and determine absorbance at 443 nm.

6. Nonenzymatic glycation (NEG) is determined as follows:
$$NEG = (NEG + EG) - EG$$

### Enzymatic Glycation

1. For determination of enzymatic glycation (EG), 0.1 mL NaOH (0.01 N) containing 400 molar excess of $NaBH_4$ is used.

2. After reduction, the glycation level is determined by the same process as mentioned above.

## Observation

| S. no. | Absorbance of control | Absorbance of test | Absorbance of standard |
|--------|----------------------|--------------------|------------------------|
| 1. | | | |
| 2. | | | |
| 3. | | | |

**Calculation:** The percentage inhibition of glycation is calculated as follows:

$$\% \text{ inhibition of glycation} = \frac{(\text{Abs control} - \text{Abs sample})}{\text{Abs control}} \times 100$$

where,   Abs control—absorbance of control
        Abs sample—absorbance of sample

## Bibliography

1. Nowotny, K, Jung, T, Höhn, A, Weber, D, and Grune, T (2015). Advanced glycation end products and oxidative stress in type 2 diabetes mellitus. Biomolecules, 5(1), 194–222.

2. Vlassara, H, and Uribarri, J (2014). Advanced glycation end products (AGE) and diabetes: cause, effect, or both?. Current Diabetes Reports, 14(1), 1–10.

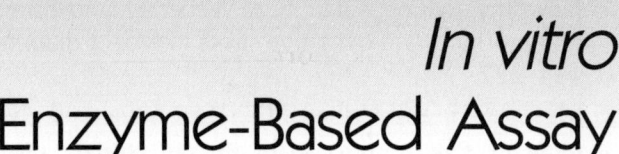

CHAPTER 5

# In vitro
# Enzyme-Based Assay

Certain enzymes are important molecular targets for drug discovery and many drug discovery programs include enzyme targets in primary screening assays. Generally, these assays utilize partially purified or purified human enzymes and involve the measurement of product formation by a variety of assay methods including radiometric, colorimetric, and fluorometric assays. Enzyme assays are performed to serve two different purposes:

i.  To identify a special enzyme, to prove its presence or absence in a distinct specimen, like an organism or a tissue.

ii.  To determine the amount of the enzyme in the sample.

While for the first, the qualitative approach, a clear positive or negative result is sufficient, the second, the quantitative approach, must deliver data as exact as possible. A great advantage of enzymes is that they can be identified by their catalysed reactions, in contrast to the other components of the cell, like functional proteins or nucleic acids, which must be determined by direct detection. During the enzyme reaction product accumulates in amounts exceeding by far the intrinsic enzyme concentration. However, the conclusion from the product formed back to the amount of enzyme in the sample comprises various difficulties and pitfalls.

## Bibliography

1. Protein-binding assays in biological liquids using microscale thermophoresis. Nature Communications, 1(7): 100. Bibcode:2010.

2. Sueyoshi, D, Anraku, Y, Komatsu, T, Urano, Y, and Kataoka, K (2017). Enzyme-Loaded Polyion Complex Vesicles as *in Vivo* Nanoreactors Working Sustainably under the Blood Circulation: Characterization and Functional Evaluation. Biomacromolecules, 18(4), 1189–1196.

## EXPERIMENT 5.1

**Aim:** To study the *in vitro* protease inhibitory potential of the given sample using protease inhibition assay.

**Principle:** Proteases or proteinases are the proteolytic enzymes which play a vital role in the normal physiological functions of cells, e.g. protein maturation, digestion, blood coagulation, control of blood pressure, immune response, etc. A variety of diseases such as cancer, pulmonary emphysema, muscular dystrophy, arthritis, pancreatitis, etc. are associated with the excessive activity of proteases. The role of proteases in diseases therefore provides targets for the possible treatment of a wide range of diseases by protease inhibitors as therapeutic agents from natural sources.

Specific and selective protease inhibitors are potentially powerful tools for inactivating target proteases in the pathogenic process of human diseases such as emphysema, arthritis, pancreatitis, thrombosis, high blood pressure, muscular dystrophy, cancer and AIDS. Protease inhibitors are one of the prime candidates with highly proven inhibitory activity against insect pests and are also known to improve the nutritional quality of food. Insects that feed on plant material possess alkaline guts and depend predominantly on serine proteases for digestion of food materials and, therefore, protease inhibitors by virtue of their antinutritional interaction can be employed effectively as defense tools. Microbial food spoilage is an area of global concern as it has been estimated that as much as 25% of all food produced is lost postharvest owing to microbial activity.

The use of an adequate amount of natural protease inhibitors is an effective way to extend the shelf life of many types of seafood such as salted fish products. This is due to the fact that the inhibitors can retard several deteriorative processes like protein degradation caused by the action of endogenous and exogenous proteases, during the food processing and preservation. Hence, protease inhibitors continue to attract the attention of researchers due to their increasing use in medicine and biotechnology.

Chromogenic substrates of proteases have a specific amino acid sequence linked to a chromophore such as *p*-nitroaniline. The action of a specific protease on its substrate causes the release of the chromophore which is measured as increase in absorbance in a recording spectrophotometer. Therefore, the amount of chromophore liberated is proportional to the activity of the enzyme. Protease inhibitor unit is defined as the amount of protease inhibitor that inhibited one unit of respective enzyme activity. Protease inhibitor activity of the respective enzyme is finally expressed in terms of percent inhibition for comparative purposes.

## Requirements

*Chemicals:* Test sample, tyrosine, casein, phosphate buffer (pH 7), Tris HCl buffer (pH 7.4), and trichloroacetic acid.

*Equipment:* UV-visible spectrophotometer and centrifuge.

*Glasswares:* Test tubes, pipettes, measuring cylinder and glass rod.

## Procedure

1. Prepare 1 mL aliquot of trypsin in 0.1 M phosphate buffer (pH 7) pre-incubated with 1 mL of a suitable dilution of the protease inhibitor at 37°C for 15 minutes.
2. To the above mixture add 2 mL of 1% casein (prepared in 0.1 M phosphate buffer) and incubated at 37°C for 30 minutes.
3. Terminate the reaction by the addition of 2.5 mL of 0.44 M trichloroacetic acid (TCA) solution.
4. Transfer the reaction mixture to a centrifuge tube and remove the precipitated protein centrifugation at 10,000 rpm for 15 minutes.
5. Measure absorbance of the clear supernatant at 280 nm in a UV-visible spectrophotometer against appropriate blanks.
6. The protease inhibitor activity is expressed in terms of percent inhibition and are quantified by comparing with tyrosine as standard.

## Alternatives

- Effect of protease inhibitor on proteases with therapeutic importance.
- Effect of sample protease inhibitor on chymotrypsin, thrombin, elastase, cathepsin-B, papain, and collagenase activities can be determined as described below:
   a. Cathespin-B activity is assayed using 1.25–2.5 units/mL of cathepsin B in cold deionised water, using 20 mM N-succinyl-Ala-Ala-Pro-Phe-P-nitroanilide in dimethyl sulphoxide as substrate at 30°C for 5 minutes. One unit of enzyme will release one micromole of *p*-nitroaniline per min from N-succinyl-Ala-Ala-Pro-Phe-*p*-nitroanilide at pH 7 at 30°C.
   b. Thrombin activity of protease inhibitor is evaluated using 1 mg/mL of thrombin in 0.1 M Tris-HCl buffer pH 7.5 and 1% Hammerstein casein as substrate at 37°C for 30 minutes.
   c. Elastase activity is tested using 10 µg/mL of elastase solution according to Kunitz caseinolytic method.
   d. Collagenase activity is assayed using 1 mg/mL of collagenase and 1% gelatin as substrate at 37°C for 30 minutes.

e. Papain activity is evaluated by caseinolytic method using papain (6 mg/mL) and 1% Hammerstein casein as substrate at 37°C for 30 minutes. The reaction is interrupted by adding 1.5 mL of TCA (5% w/v).

f. Chymotrypsin activity is assayed by dissolving in 0.05 M Tris-HCl buffer, (pH 7.6), 20 mM peptide substrate, N-succinyl-Ala-Ala-Pro-Phe-P-nitroanilide, 0.27 mg/mL of inhibitor and chymotrypsin (10 µg/mL). One unit of enzyme is defined as the amount of enzyme that resulted in the conversion of 1 µmol substrate per minute.

## Observation

| S. no. | Absorbance of control | Absorbance of test | Absorbance of standard |
|--------|----------------------|--------------------|------------------------|
| 1. | | | |
| 2. | | | |
| 3. | | | |

**Calculation:** The percentage inhibition of protease is calculated as follows:

$$\% \text{ inhibition of protease} = \frac{(\text{Abs control} - \text{Abs sample})}{\text{Abs control}} \times 100$$

where, Abs control—absorbance of control

Abs sample—absorbance of sample

where, $V_0$—volume of $Na_2S_2O_3$ solution used to titrate the control mixture

$V_1$—titrated volume of the mixture containing the samples

## Bibliography

1. Bronstein, I, Voyta, J, Palmer, M, and Tillotson, B (2001). US Patent No. 6,243,980. Washington, DC: US Patent and Trademark Office.

2. Neves, AC, Harnedy, PA, O'Keeffe, MB, and FitzGerald, RJ (2017). Bioactive peptides from Atlantic salmon (Salmo salar) with angiotensin converting enzyme and dipeptidyl peptidase IV inhibitory, and antioxidant activities. Food Chemistry, 218, 396–405.

**EXPERIMENT 5.2**

**Aim:** To study the *in vitro* tyrosinase inhibitory potential of the given sample using tyrosinase inhibition assay.

**Principle:** Tyrosinase is an enzyme responsible for the synthesis of dermal melanin pigment from L-tyrosine and L-dihydroxyphenylalanine (L-DOPA) within the melanocytes on the melanosomes. It has several functions including hydroxylation of L-tyrosine and oxidation of L-DOPA to dopaquinone and subsequent autopolymerization to melanin. The over-production of melanin has been associated with the condition of hyperpigmentation of skin such as melasma and ephelides. Therefore, the inhibition of tyrosinase enzyme is reflective of controlling hyper-pigmentation and associated conditions. Tyrosinase first hydroxylates L-tyrosine to L-DOPA and then oxidizes L-DOPA to dopaquinone which is subsequently converted to dopachrome. The activity of tyrosinase enzyme is proportional to the amount of dopachrome liberated that is measured at 475 nm in a spectrophotometer.

### Requirements

*Chemicals:* Test sample, L-tyrosine, L-DOPA, and phosphate buffer (pH 7).

*Equipment:* UV-visible spectrophotometer.

*Glasswares:* Test tubes, pipettes, measuring cylinder and glass rod.

### Procedure

1. Dispense 1.0 mL of phosphate buffer is in a test tube.
2. Add 500 µL of tyrosinase enzyme solution and 500 µL of test sample. Mix and incubate.
3. Finally add 1.0 mL substrate solution (2.55 mM L-DOPA or 1.75 mM L-tyrosine prepared in phosphate buffer) and measure absorbance at 475 nm.

### Observation

| S. no. | Absorbance of control | Absorbance of test | Absorbance of standard |
|--------|----------------------|--------------------|-----------------------|
| 1. | | | |
| 2. | | | |
| 3. | | | |

**Calculation:** The percentage inhibition of tyrosine is calculated as follows:

$$\% \text{ inhibition of tyrosine} = \frac{(\text{Abs control} - \text{Abs sample})}{\text{Abs control}} \times 100$$

where, Abs control—absorbance of control

Abs sample—absorbance of sample

## Bibliography

1. Druker, BJ, Tamura, S, Buchdunger, E, Ohno, S, Segal, GM, Fanning, S, and Lydon, NB (1996). Effects of a selective inhibitor of the Abl tyrosine kinase on the growth of Bcr-Abl positive cells. Nature Medicine, 2(5), 561–566.

2. Rusnak, DW, Lackey, K, Affleck, K, Wood, ER, Alligood, KJ, Rhodes, N, and Gilmer, TM (2001). The effects of the novel, reversible epidermal growth factor receptor/ErbB-2 tyrosine kinase inhibitor, GW2016, on the growth of human normal and tumor-derived cell lines *in vitro* and *in vivo*. Molecular Cancer Therapeutics, 1(2), 85–94.

**Aim:** To study the *in vitro* acetylcholinesterases (AChE) inhibitory potential of the given sample using acetylcholinesterases inhibition assay.

**Principle:** Acetylcholinesterase plays an important role in the central and peripheral nervous systems, along with the acetylcholine receptor, in the transmission of action potential across nerve-nerve and neuromuscular synapses. The enzyme's physiological task is the hydrolytic destruction of the cationic neurotransmitter, acetylcholine.

Because of the pivotal role that acetylcholinesterase plays in the nervous system, it has long been an attractive target for the rational design and discovery of mechanism based inhibitors. Some inhibitors of acetylcholinesterase are known to be useful for the treatment of Alzheimer's disease, senile dementia, ataxia and for improving the long-term memory processes by enhancing cholinergic activity.

The principle involves the measurements of the rate of production of thiocholine, as acetylthiocholine is hydrolyzed by acetylcholinesterase. Hydrolysis of acetylthiocholine is accompanied by a continuous reaction between the thiocholine liberated and dithiobisnitrobenzoic acid (DTNB) which produces the yellow anion of 5-thio-2-nitrobenzoic acid. The rate of anion production is measured from the absorbance at 412 nm.

### Requirements

*Chemicals:* Test sample, phosphate buffer saline, 5,5′-dithio-bis (2-nitrobenzoic acid) (DTNB), acetylcholinestrase, galanthamine, Tris-HCl buffer pH 8.0 and distilled water.

*Equipment:* UV-visible spectrophotometer.

*Glasswares:* Test tubes, micropipettes, measuring cylinder and glass rod.

### Procedure

1. In the test tube add 1000 µL of 50 mM Tris-HCl buffer pH 8.0 and 250 µL of test sample at the concentrations of 25–400 µg/mL, 10 µL, 6.67 µmL$^{-1}$ AChE and 20 µL of 10 mM of DTNB in buffer.

2. Prepare positive control, namely galanthamine in serial concentration as same as test sample by dissolving in 50 mM Tris-HCl buffer pH 8.0.

3. Incubate the mixture for 15 minutes at 37°C. Then add 10 µL of acetylthiocholine iodide (200 mM) in buffer to the mixture and measure absorbance at 412 nm every 10 seconds for 3 minutes, for a blank use buffer instead of enzyme solution.

## Observation

| S. no. | Absorbance of control | Absorbance of test | Absorbance of standard |
|---|---|---|---|
| 1. | | | |
| 2. | | | |
| 3. | | | |

**Calculation:** The percentage inhibition of acetylcholinestrase is calculated as follows:

$$\% \text{ inhibition of acetylcholinestrase} = \frac{(\text{Abs control} - \text{Abs sample})}{\text{Abs control}} \times 100$$

where, Abs control—absorbance of control

Abs sample—absorbance of sample

## Bibliography

1. Vinutha, B, Prashanth, D, Salma, K, Sreeja, SL, Pratiti, D, Padmaja, R, and Deepak, M (2007). Screening of selected Indian medicinal plants for acetylcholinesterase inhibitory activity. Journal of Ethnopharmacology, 109(2), 359–363.

2. Wang, M, Gu, X, Zhang, G, Zhang, D, and Zhu, D (2009). Continuous colorimetric assay for acetylcholinesterase and inhibitor screening with gold nanoparticles. Langmuir, 25(4), 2504–2507.

# CHAPTER 6

# In vitro Antimicrobial Assay

*Chemotherapy* is the term originally used to describe the use of drugs that are 'selectively toxic' to invading microorganisms while having minimal effects on the host. All living organisms are prey to infection. Humans, being no exception to this rule, are susceptible to diseases caused by viruses, bacteria, protozoa, fungi and helminths.

Antimicrobial drugs have the greatest contribution of the 20th century to therapeutics. Their advent changed the outlook of the physician about the power drugs can have on diseases. They are one of the few curative drugs. Their importance is magnified in the developing countries like India, where infective diseases predominate. As a class, they are one of the most frequently used as well as misused drugs. The use of chemotherapeutic agents dates back to the work of Ehrlich and others and to the development of arsenical drugs such as salvarsan for the treatment of syphilis.

The inevitable consequence of their widespread use has been the emergence of antibiotic-resistant pathogens, fueling an ever-increasing need for new drugs at a time when the pace of antimicrobial drug development has slowed dramatically. Reducing inappropriate antibiotic use is thought to be the best way to control resistance. Antimicrobial susceptibility tests are used to determine which specific antibiotics a particular bacteria or fungus is sensitive to. Most often, this testing complements a Gram stain and culture, the results of which are obtained much sooner.

## Bibliography

1. Birger, RB, Kouyos, RD, Cohen, T, Griffiths, EC, Huijben, S, Mina, MJ and Metcalf, CJE (2015). The potential impact of coinfection on antimicrobial chemotherapy and drug resistance. Trends in Microbiology, 23(9), 537–544.

2. Feazel, LM, Malhotra, A, Perencevich, EN, Kaboli, P, Diekema, DJ, and Schweizer, ML (2014). Effect of antibiotic stewardship programmes on Clostridium difficile incidence: a systematic review and meta-analysis. Journal of Antimicrobial Chemotherapy, 69(7), 1748–1754.

## CULTURE MEDIA

Microorganisms need nutrients, a source of energy and certain environmental conditions in order to grow and reproduce. In the environment, microbes have adapted to the habitats most suitable for their needs, in the laboratory, however, these requirements must be met by a culture medium. This is basically an aqueous solution to which all the necessary nutrients have been added. Depending on the type and combination of nutrients, different categories of media can be made.

### Types of Culture Media

A growth medium or a culture medium is defined as the solid or liquid formulation which contains the nutrients and other necessary materials to support the growth of microorganisms and cells. Media are predominantly classified on the basis of consistency and chemical composition. Based on consistency, growth media can be classified as growth media can be either solid or liquid preparations.

### *Solid Media*

Most culture media are prepared as solid formulations by adding a solidification agent (agar) generally at the concentration of 1.5%. Agar is a jelly-like substance which is used to solidify the medium. It is an inert substance which does not have a nutritional value. Agar is extracted from several species of red algae. The commercial agar is derived mainly from Gelidium red algae. Solid medium is a mixture of agar and other nutrients. When agar is added, the medium becomes solid at room temperature.

### Advantages of solid media:

1. Bacteria may be identified by studying the colony character.
2. Mixed bacteria can be separated. Solid media is used for the isolation of bacteria as pure culture. 'Agar' is most commonly used to prepare solid media. Agar is polysaccharide extract obtained from seaweed. Agar is an ideal solidifying agent as it is:
   a. Bacteriologically inert, i.e. no influence on bacterial growth,
   b. It remains solid at 37°C, and
   c. It is transparent.

*Liquid Media*

The key difference between solid and liquid media is that solid media contain agar while liquid media do not contain agar. It is used for profuse growth, e.g. blood culture in liquid media. Mixed organisms cannot be separated.

On the basis of composition growth media is further classified as routine laboratory and synthetic media. The routine laboratory media is further divided into basal media, enriched media, selective media, indicator media, transport media, and storage media. A brief description of the routine media is given below:

1. *Basal media*: Basal media are those that may be used for growth (culture) of bacteria that do not need enrichment of the media. *Examples*: Nutrient broth, nutrient agar, and peptone water. Staphylococcus and Enterobacteriaceae grow in these media.

2. *Enriched media*: The media are enriched usually by adding blood, serum or egg. *Examples*: Enriched media are blood agar and Lowenstein-Jensen media. Streptococci grow in blood agar media.

3. *Selective media*: These media favour the growth of a particular bacterium by inhibiting the growth of undesired bacteria and allowing growth of desirable bacteria. *Examples*: MacConkey agar, Lowenstein-Jensen media, tellurite media (tellurite inhibits the growth of most of the throat organisms except diphtheria bacilli). Antibiotic may be added to a medium for inhibition.

4. *Indicator (differential) media*: An indicator is included in the medium. A particular organism causes change in the indicator, e.g. blood, neutral red, tellurite. *Examples*: Blood agar and MacConkey agar are indicator media.

5. *Transport media*: These media are used when specimen cannot be cultured soon after collection. *Examples*: Cary-Blair medium, amies medium, Stuart medium.

6. *Storage media*: Media used for storing the bacteria for a long period of time. *Examples*: Egg saline medium, chalk cooked meat broth.

**Some commonly employed synthetic media are discussed below:**

*Nutrient broth media:* 500 g meat, e.g. ox heart is minced and mixed with 1 litre water. 10 g peptone and 5 g sodium chloride are added, pH is adjusted to 7.3.

*Uses:* (1) As a basal media for the preparation of other media. (2) To study soluble products of bacteria.

*Nutrient agar media:* It is solid at 37°C. 2.5% agar is added in nutrient broth. It is heated at 100°C to melt the agar and then cooled.

Plate 1

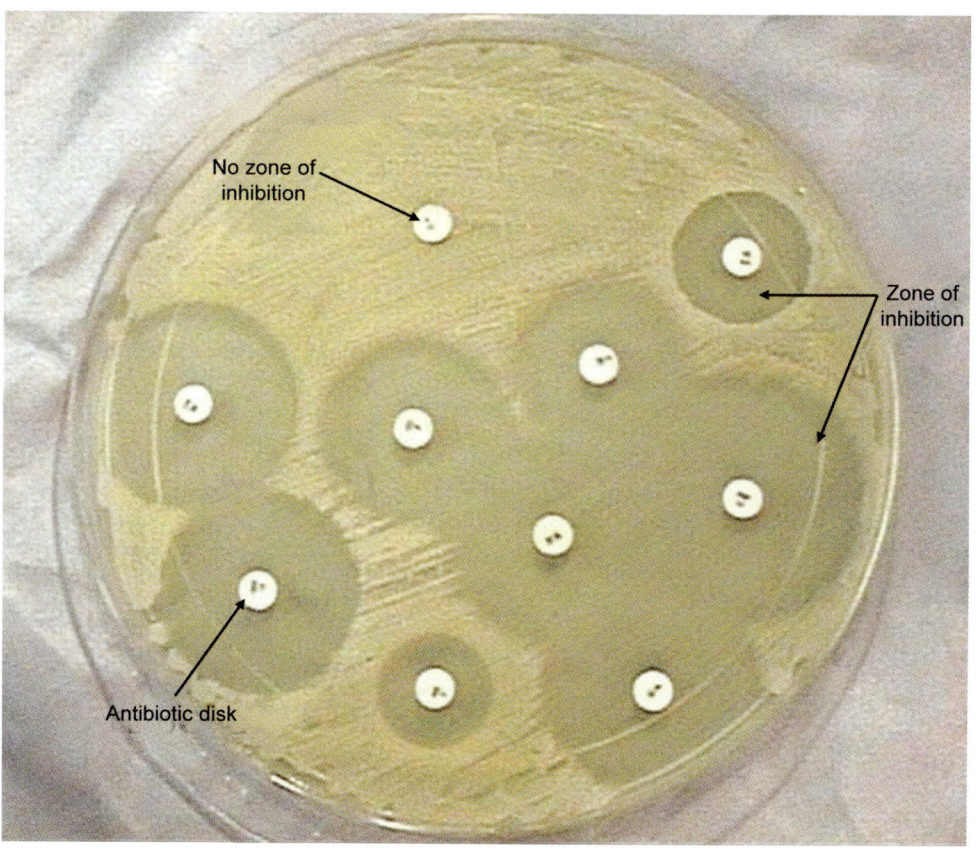

**Fig. 6.1:** Antibiotic sensitivity test by Kirby-Bauer method

Plate 2

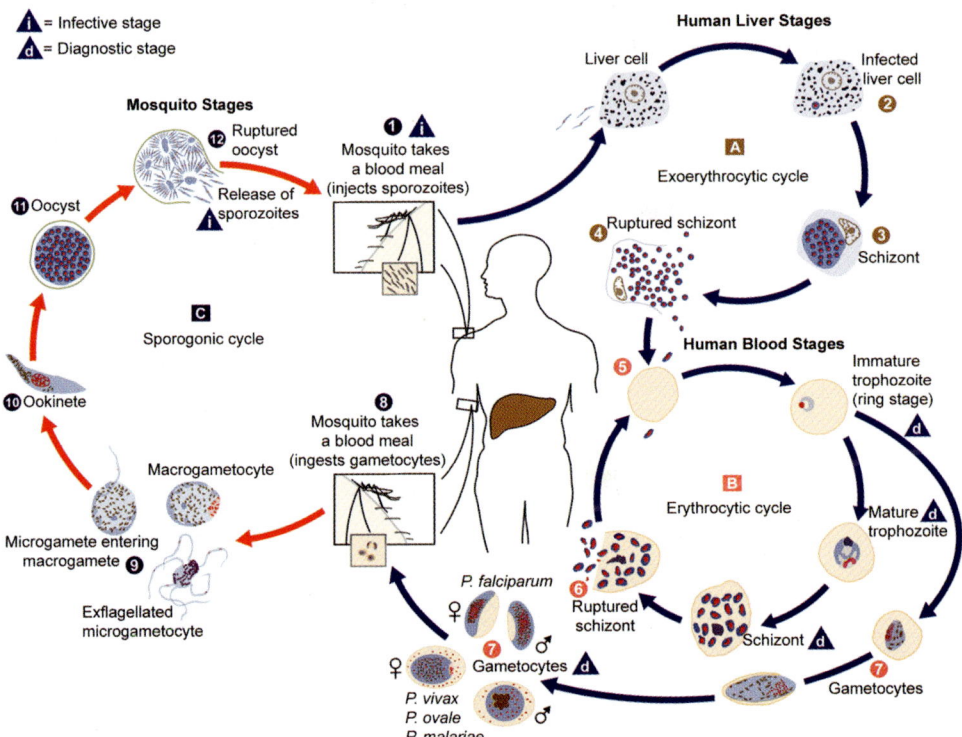

**Fig. 7.1:** Life cycle of malarial parasite both in host and vector. The malaria parasite life cycle involves two hosts. During a blood meal, a malaria-infected female Anopheles mosquito inoculates sporozoites into the human host (1), sporozoites infect liver cells (2) and mature into schizonts, which rupture and release merozoites (4). Of note, in *P. vivax* and *P. ovale* a dormant stage (hypnozoites) can persist in the liver and cause relapses by invading the bloodstream weeks, or even years later.) After this initial replication in the liver (exoerythrocytic schizogony) (A), the parasites undergo asexual multiplication in the erythrocytes (erythrocytic schizogony) (B). Merozoites infect red blood cells (5). The ring stage trophozoites mature into schizonts, which rupture releasing merozoites (5). Some parasites differentiate into sexual erythrocytic stages (gametocytes) (7). Blood stage parasites are responsible for the clinical manifestations of the disease. The gametocytes, male (microgametocytes) and female (macrogametocytes), are ingested by an Anopheles mosquito during a blood meal (8). The parasites' multiplication in the mosquito is known as the sporogonic cycle (C). While in the mosquito's stomach, the microgametes penetrate the macrogametes generating zygotes (9). The zygotes in turn become motile and elongated (ookinetes) (10) which invade the midgut wall of the mosquito where they develop into oocysts (11). The oocysts grow, rupture, and release sporozoites (12), which make their way to the mosquito's salivary glands. Inoculation of the sporozoites (1) into a new human host perpetuates the malaria life cycle.

Plate 3

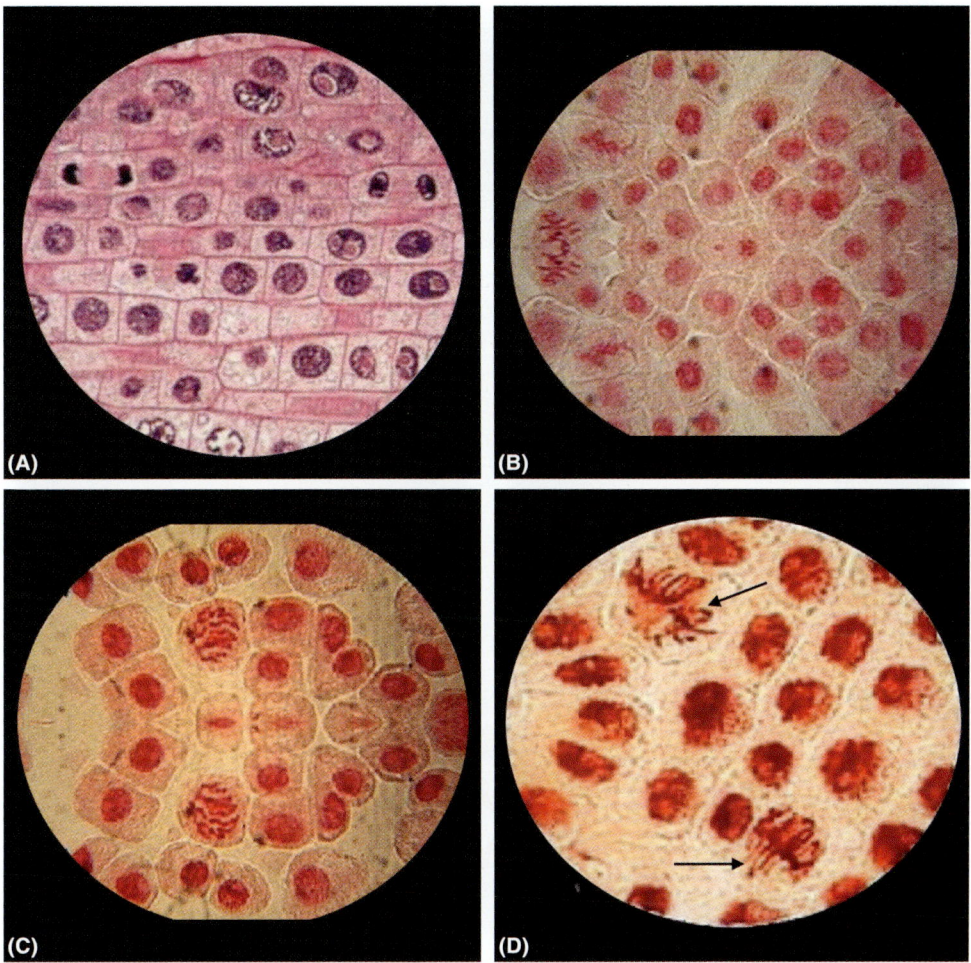

**Fig. 8.1A to D:** *Allium cepa* root meristem cells in mitotic dividing stage (Patel et al., 2013). (A) Normal cells in telophase mitotic dividing stage; (B and C) abnormal dividing cells in standard drug treated group showing multipolarity and sticky chromosome; (D) normal as well as few abnormal dividing cells in test treated root showing sticky and vagrant chromosome.

Plate 4

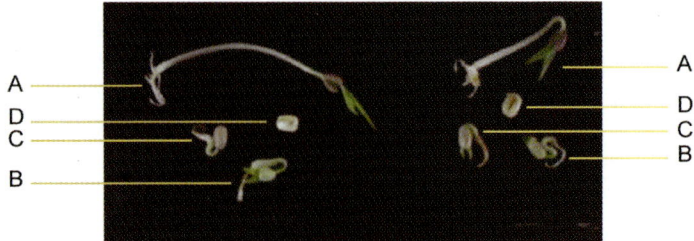

**Fig. 8.2:** Germination of green-gram seeds in water in the presence and absence of test sample is shown in the figure. The sprouted seed had developed roots, shoot and two leaves (A). In contrast, seeds that sprouted in the presence of 10 µL test sample had reduced growth with shortened shoot and small leaves (B), with no visible roots. At 20 µL concentration inhibition of growth was much more pronounced, and at 100 µL, inhibition of germination was complete with no visible sprouting (C and D). These morphological observations indicate the dose dependence of inhibition. (Murthy et al., 2011).

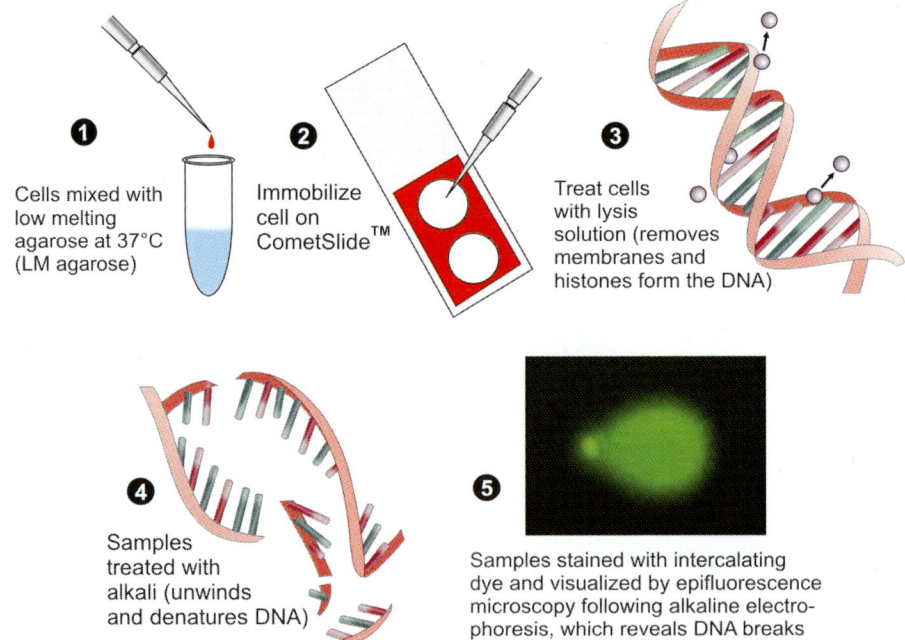

**Fig. 8.4:** Diagrammatic representation of Comet assay procedure and anticipated result
1. Cells are mixed with low melting point agarose.
2. Immobilised on CometSlide™.
3. Cells are lysed to remove membranes and DNA associated proteins before alkaline treatment to unwind and denature DNA.
4. During electrophoresis, damaged, unwound, relaxed DNA migrates out of the cell and can be visualized using fluorescent dye (For e.g. SYBR® Green).

Plate 5

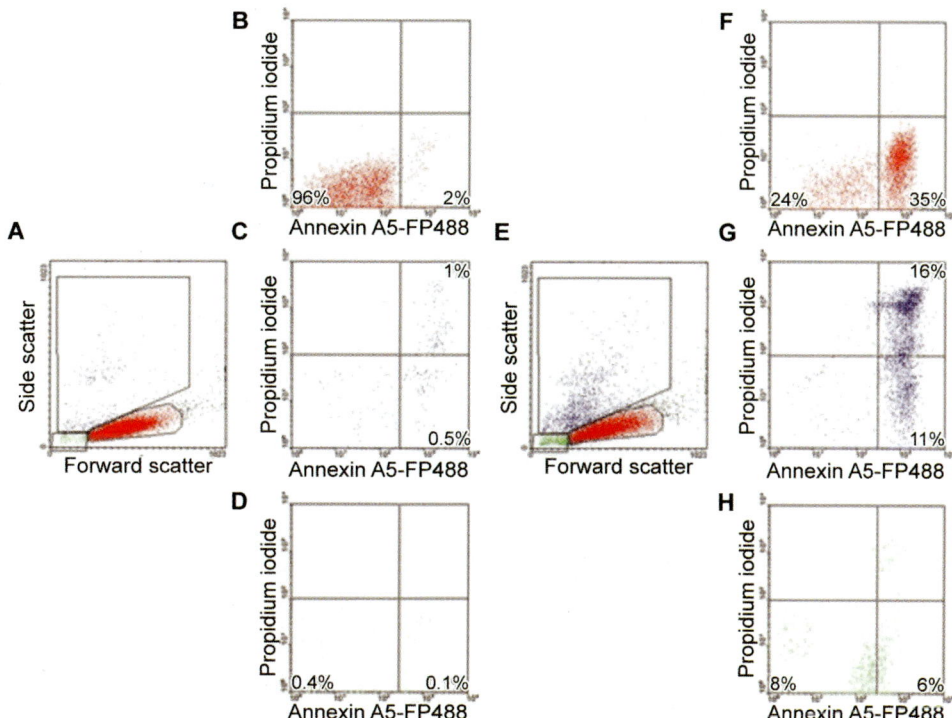

**Fig. 8.5:** Flow cytometry of apoptotic Jurkat cells with annexin A5-FP488 and propidium iodide. Forward- and side-scatter plots of untreated control Jurkat cells (A) and Jurkat cells treated with antibody to Fas (E). (B–D,F–H) Annexin A5-FP488 and propidium iodide dot plots of living and early apoptotic cells (red; B, F), dot plots of dead cells with compromised integrity of the plasma membrane (blue; C, G) and dot plots of apoptotic bodies (green; D, H). Bottom left quadrants, living cells; bottom right quadrants, cells in the early phase of cell death; top right quadrants, cells in the phase of cell death with leaky plasma membrane

Plate 6

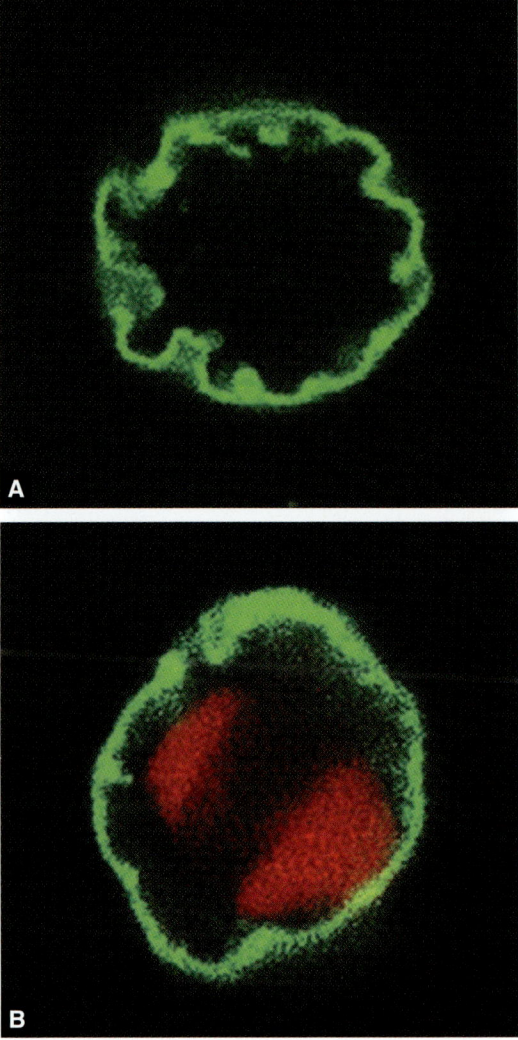

**Fig. 8.6A and B:** CSLM analysis of apoptotic Jurkat cells with annexin A5-FP488 and propidium iodide. Images are of an early apoptotic Jurkat cell (A) and a late apoptotic Jurkat cell with a leaky plasma membrane (B). Original magnification, X63.

Plate 7

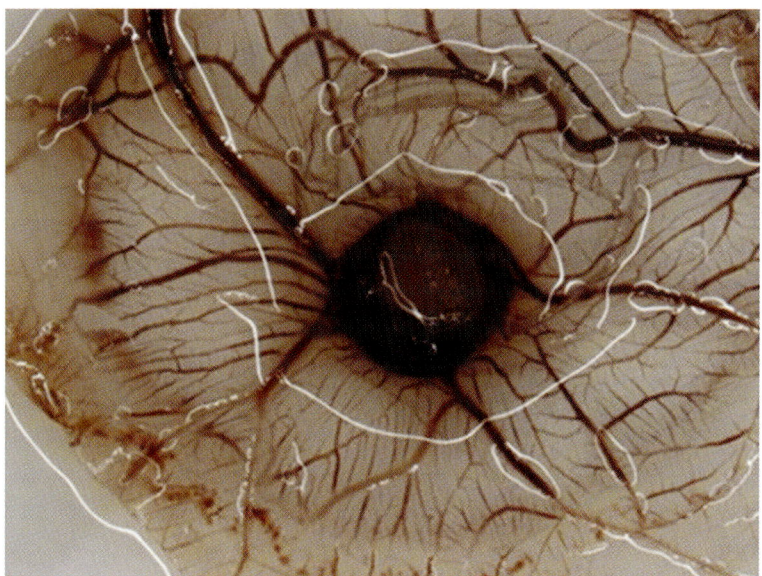

**Fig. 8.10:** The vascular zone of the CAM

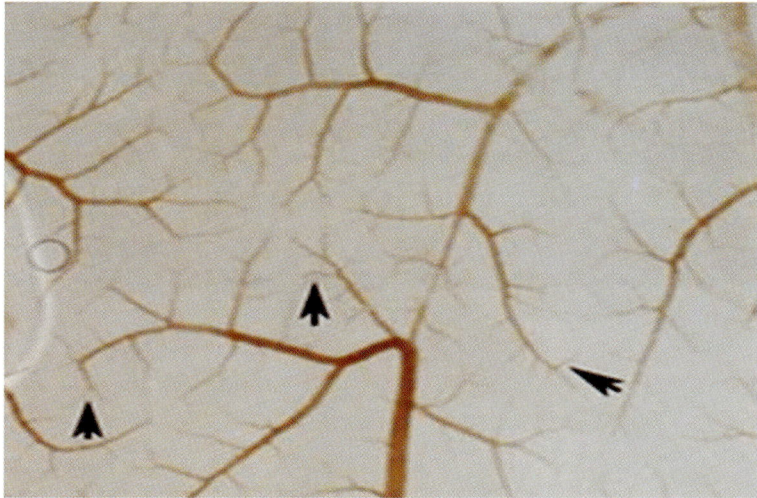

**Fig. 8.11:** Blood vessel branch points on CAM (arrow indicates new-formed blood vessel branches)

Plate 8

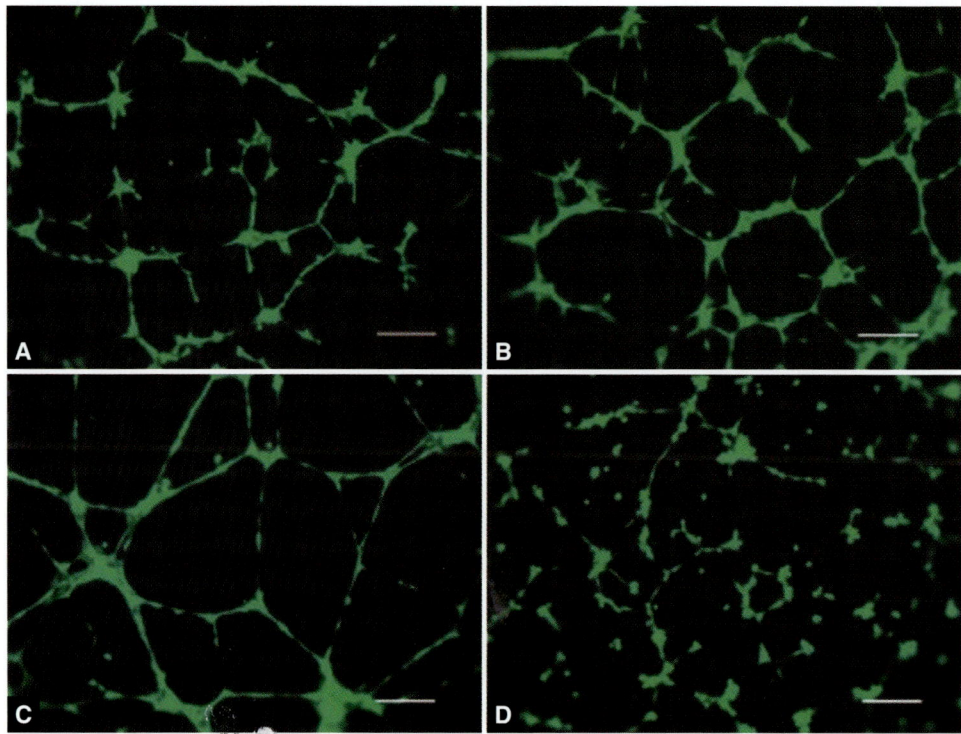

**Fig. 8.12A and B:** Effect of angiogenesis stimulators and an inhibitor on tube formation. Shown is the appearance of endothelial cell tubes on a basement membrane substratum in the (A) endothelial basal media-2 (EBM-2) without angiogenesis stimulators; (B) EBM-2 with 10 mM bFGF; (C) endothelial growth media (EGM-2) that contains 2% fetal bovine serum, hydrocortisone, bFGF, VEGF, R3-IGF, ascorbic acid, heparin, hEGF and GA-1000; and in the (D) EGM-2 with 15 μM of sulforaphane, an inhibitor of angiogenensis

*Peptone water media:* Peptone 1% and sodium chloride 0.5%. It is used as base for sugar media and to test indole formation.

*Blood agar media:* Most commonly used medium. 5–10% defibrinated sheep or horse blood is added to melted agar at 45–50°C. Blood acts as an enrichment material and also as an indicator. Certain bacteria when grown in blood agar produce hemolysis around their colonies. Certain bacteria produce no hemolysis. Based on the types of changes the type of organism infecting the blood sample can be detected. For example:

- The colony is surrounded by a clear zone of complete hemolysis, called beta (β) hemolysis, e.g. *Streptococcus pyogenes* is a beta hemolytic streptococci.
- The colony is surrounded by a zone of greenish discoloration due to formation of biliverdin, is alpha (α) hemolysis, e.g. viridans streptococci,
- Gamma (γ) hemolysis, is media without hemolysis. There is no change in the medium surrounding the colony.

*Chocolate agar or heated blood agar media:* Prepared by heating blood agar. It is used for culture of pneumococcus, gonococcus, meningococcus and hemophilus. Heating the blood inactivates inhibitor of growths.

*MacConkey agar media:* Most commonly used for E terobacteriaceae. It contains agar, peptone, sodium chloride, bile salt, lactose and neutral red. It is a selective and indicator medium:

1. Selective as bile salt does not inhibit the growth of Enterobactericeae but inhibits growth of many other bacteria.
2. Indicator medium as the colonies of bacteria that ferment lactose take a pink color due to production of acid. Acid turns the indicator neutral red to pink. These bacteria are called 'lactose fermenter', e.g. *Escherichia coli*. Colorless colony indicates that lactose is not fermented, i.e. the bacterium is nonlactose fermenter, e.g. Salmonella, Shigella, and Vibrio.

*Müeller-Hinton agar media:* Disc diffusion sensitivity tests for antimicrobial drugs should be carried out on this media as per WHO recommendation to promote reproducibility and comparability of results.

*Hiss serum water medium:* This medium is used to study the fermentation reactions of bacteria which cannot grow in peptone water sugar media, e.g. pneumococcus, Neisseria, and Corynebacterium.

*Lowenstein-Jensen medium:* It is used to culture tubercle bacilli. It contains egg, malachite green, and glycerol. (1) Egg is an enrichment material which stimulates the growth of tubercle bacilli. (2) Malachite green inhibits growth of organisms other than mycobacteria. (3) Glycerol promotes the growth of *Mycobacterium tuberculosis* but not *Mycobacterium bovis*.

***Dubos medium:*** This liquid medium is used for tubercle bacilli. In this medium drug sensitivity of tubercle bacilli can be carried out. It contains 'tween 80', bovine serum albumin, casein hydrolysate, asparagin and salts. Tween 80 causes dispersed growth and bovine albumin causes rapid growth.

***Loeffler serum:*** Serum is used for enrichment. Diphtheria bacilli grow in this medium in 6 hours when the secondary bacteria do not grow. It is used for rapid diagnosis of diphtheria and to demonstrate volutin granules. It contains sheep, ox or horse serum.

***Tellurite blood agar:*** It is used as a selective medium for isolation of *Corynebacterium diphtheriae*. Tellurite inhibits the growth of most secondary bacteria without an inhibitory effect on diphtheria bacilli. It is also an indicator medium as the diphtheria bacilli produce black colonies. Tellurite metabolized to tellbrism, which has black color.

***Eosin-methylene blue (EMB) agar:*** A selective and differential medium for enteric gram-negative rods. Lactose-fermenting colonies are colored and nonlactose-fermenting colonies are nonpigmented. Selects against gram-positive bacteria.

***Xylose lysine deoxycholate (XLD):*** It is used to isolate Salmonella and Shigella species from stool specimens. This is a selective media.

***Salmonella-Shigella (SS) agar:*** It is a selective medium used to isolate Salmonella and Shigella species. SS agar with additional bile salt is used if *Yersinia enterocolitica* is suspected.

***Deoxycholate citrate agar (DCA):*** It is used for isolation of Salmonella and Shigella. The other enteric bacteria are mostly inhibited (a selective medium). It is also a differential (indicator) medium due to presence of lactose and neutral red.

***Tetrathionate broth:*** This medium is used for isolating Salmonella from stool. It acts as a selective medium. It inhibits normal intestinal bacteria and permits multiplication of Salmonella.

***Selenite F broth:*** Uses and functions are same as that of tetrathionate broth.

***Thiosulphate-citrate-bile-sucrose (TCBS) agar:*** TCBS agar is a selective medium used to isolate *Vibrio cholerae* and other Vibrio species from stool.

***Charcoal-yeast agar:*** Used for *Legionella pneumophila*. Increased concentration of iron and cysteine allows growth.

***Tellurite-gelatin agar medium (TGAM):*** It may be used as transport, selective and indicator medium.

***Campylobacter medium:*** This selective medium is used to isolate *Campylobacter jejuni* and *Campylobacter coli* from stool.

***Cary-Blair medium:*** It is used as a transport medium for feces that may contain Salmonella, Shigella, Vibrio or Campylobacter species.

Amies medium is used for gonococci and other pathogens.

***Peptone water sugar media:*** These indicator media are used to study 'sugar fermentation'. 1% solution of a sugar (lactose, glucose, mannitol, etc.) is added to peptone water containing Andrade's indicator in a test tube. A small inverted Durham tube is placed in the medium. The media are colorless. After culture, change of a medium to red color indicates acid production. Gas, if produced, collects in Durham tube.

***Motility indole urea (MIU) medium:*** This is used to differentiate enterobacteria species by their motility, urease, and indole reactions.

***Kligler iron agar (KIA):*** This is a differential slope medium used in the identification of enteric bacteria. The reactions are based on the fermentation of lactose and glucose and the production of hydrogen sulphide.

***Christensen's urea medium:*** This is used to identify urea splitting organisms, e.g. Proteus. A purple pink colour indicates urea splitting.

***Bordet-Gengou medium:*** This medium is used for culture of *Bordetella pertussis*. Increased concentration of blood allows growth. It contains agar, potato, sodium chloride, glycerol, peptone and 50% horse blood. Penicillin may be added to it.

A chemically-defined (synthetic) medium (Tables 6.1 and 6.2) is one in which the exact chemical composition is known. A complex (undefined) medium is one in which the exact chemical constitution of the medium is not known. Defined media are usually composed of pure biochemicals off the shelf; complex media usually contain complex materials of biological origin such as blood or milk or yeast extract or beef extract, the exact chemical composition of which is obviously undetermined. A defined medium is a minimal medium if it provides only the exact nutrients (including any growth factors) needed by the organism for growth. The use of defined minimal media requires the investigator to know the exact nutritional requirements of the organisms in question. Chemically-defined media are of value in studying the minimal nutritional requirements of microorganisms, for enrichment cultures, and for a wide variety of physiological studies. Complex media usually provide the full range of

**Table 6.1:** Minimal medium for the growth of *Bacillus megaterium*. An example of a chemically-defined medium for growth of a heterotrophic bacterium

| Component | Amount | Function of component |
|---|---|---|
| Sucrose | 10.0 g | C and energy source |
| $K_2HPO_4$ | 2.5 g | pH buffer; P and K source |
| $KH_2PO_4$ | 2.5 g | pH buffer; P and K source |
| $(NH_4)_2 HPO_4$ | 1.0 g | pH buffer; N and P source |
| $MgSO_4 7H_2O$ | 0.20 g | S and $Mg^{++}$ source |
| $FeSO_4 7H_2O$ | 0.01 g | $Fe^{++}$ source |
| $MnSO_4 7H_2O$ | 0.007 g | $Mn^{++}$ source |
| Water | 985 mL | |
| pH 7.0 | | |

**Table 6.2:** Defined medium for the growth of *Thiobacillus thiooxidans*, a litho-autotrophic bacterium

| Component | Amount | Function of component |
|---|---|---|
| $NH_4Cl$ | 0.52 g | N source |
| $KH_2PO_4$ | 0.28 g | P and K source |
| $MgSO_4 7H_2O$ | 0.25 g | S and $Mg^{++}$ source |
| $CaCl_2 2H_2O$ | 0.07 g | $Ca^{++}$ source |
| Elemental sulfur | 1.56 g | Energy source |
| $CO_2$ | 5%* | C source |
| Water | 1000 mL | |
| pH 3.0 | | |

*Aerate medium intermittently with air containing 5% $CO_2$.

growth factors that may be required by an organism so they may be more handily used to cultivate unknown bacteria or bacteria whose nutritional requirement are complex (i.e. organisms that require a lot of growth factors, known or unknown). Complex media are usually used for cultivation of bacterial pathogens and other fastidious bacteria.

Most pathogenic bacteria of animals, which have adapted themselves to growth in animal tissues, require complex media for their growth. Blood, serum and tissue extracts are frequently added to culture media for the cultivation of pathogens. Even so, for a few fastidious pathogens such as *Treponema pallidum*, the agent of syphilis, and *Mycobacterium leprae*, the cause of leprosy, artificial culture media and conditions have not been established. This fact thwarts the ability to do basic research on these pathogens and the diseases that they cause.

Other concepts employed in the construction of culture media are the principles of selection and enrichment. A selective medium is one which has a component(s) added to it which will inhibit or prevent the growth of certain types or species of bacteria and/or promote the growth of desired species. One can also adjust the physical conditions of a culture medium, such as pH and temperature, to render it selective for organisms that are able to grow under these certain conditions.

A culture medium may also be a differential medium if allows the investigator to distinguish between different types of bacteria based on some observable trait in their pattern of growth on the medium. Thus a selective, differential medium for the isolation of *Staphylococcus aureus*, the most common bacterial pathogen of humans, contains a very high concentration of salt (which the staph will tolerate) that inhibits most other bacteria, mannitol as a source of fermentable sugar, and a pH indicator dye. From clinical specimens, only staph will grow. *S. aureus* is differentiated from *S. epidermidis* (a nonpathogenic component of the normal flora) on the basis of its ability to ferment mannitol. Mannitol-fermenting colonies (*S. aureus*) produce acid which reacts with the indicator dye forming a colored halo around the colonies; mannitol nonfermenters (*S. epidermidis*) use other nonfermentative substrates in the medium for growth and do not form a halo around their colonies.

An enrichment medium employs a slightly different twist. An enrichment medium (Tables 6.3 and 6.4) contains some component that permits the growth of specific types or species of bacteria, usually because they alone can utilize the component from their environment. However, an enrichment medium may have selective features. An enrichment medium for nonsymbiotic nitrogen-fixing bacteria omits a source of added nitrogen to the medium. The medium is inoculated with a potential source of these bacteria (e.g. a soil sample) and incubated in the atmosphere wherein the

**Table 6.3:** Complex medium for the growth of fastidious bacteria

| Component | Amount | Function of component |
| --- | --- | --- |
| Beef extract | 1.5 g | Source of vitamins and other growth factors |
| Yeast extract | 3.0 g | Source of vitamins and other growth factors |
| Peptone | 6.0 g | Source of amino acids, N, S, and P |
| Glucose | 1.0 g | C and energy source |
| Agar | 15.0 g | Inert solidifying agent |
| Water | 1000 mL | |
| pH 6.6 | | |

**Table 6.4:** Selective enrichment medium for growth of extreme halophiles

| Component | Amount | Function of component |
|---|---|---|
| Casamino acids | 7.5 g | Source of amino acids, N, S and P |
| Yeast extract | 10.0 g | Source of growth factors |
| Trisodium citrate | 3.0 g | C and energy source |
| KCl | 2.0 g | $K^+$ source |
| $MgSO_4$ 7 $H_2O$ | 20.0 g | S and $Mg^{++}$ source |
| $FeCl_2$ | 0.023 g | $Fe^{++}$ source |
| NaCl | 250 g | $Na^+$ source for halophiles and inhibitory to nonhalophiles |
| Water | 1000 mL | |
| pH 7.4 | | |

only source of nitrogen available is $N_2$. A selective enrichment medium for growth of the extreme halophile (Halococcus) contains nearly 25% salt (NaCl), which is required by the extreme halophile and which inhibits the growth of all other prokaryotes.

## Preparation of Microbiological Culture Media

The survival and growth of microorganisms depend on available and a favorable growth environment. Culture media are nutrient solutions used in laboratories to grow microorganisms. For the successful cultivation of a given microorganism, it is necessary to understand its nutritional requirements and then supply the essential nutrients in the proper form and proportion in a culture medium. The general composition of a medium is as follows:

- H-donors and acceptors (approximately 1–15 g/L)
- C-source (approximately 1–20 g/L)
- N-source (approximately 0.2–2 g/L)
- Other inorganic nutrients, e.g. S, P (50 mg/L)
- Trace elements (0.1–1 µg/L)
- Growth factors (amino acids, purines, pyrimidines, occasionally 50 mg/L, vitamins occasionally 0.1–1 mg/L)
- Solidifying agent (e.g. agar 10–20 g/L)
- Solvent (usually distilled water)
- Buffer chemicals

Microbiological culture media as stated earlier could be classified according to:

1. *Consistency, which could be adjusted by changing the concentration of solidifying or gelling agents, e.g. agar, gelatine (liquid media do not contain such materials)*

   - Cultures in liquid media (or broth) are usually handled in tubes or flasks and incubated under static or shaken conditions. This way, homogenous conditions are generated for growth and metabolism studies, (e.g. with the control of optical density and allowing sampling for the analysis of metabolic products).

   - Semisolid media are usually used in fermentation and cell mobility studies, and are also suitable for promoting anaerobic growth.

   - Solid media are prepared in test tubes or in Petri dishes, in the latter case, the solid medium is called agar plate. In the case of tubes, medium is solidified in a slanted position, which is called agar slant, or in an upright position, which is called agar deep tube. Solid media are used to determine colony morphology, isolate cultures, enumerate and isolate bacteria (e.g. using dilutions from a mixed bacterial population in combination with spreading), and for the detection of specific biochemical reactions (e.g. metabolic activities connected with diffusing extracellular enzymes that act with insoluble substrates of the agar medium).

2. *Composition*

   - Chemically-defined (or synthetic) media are composed only of pure chemicals with defined quantity and quality.

   - Complex (or nonsynthetic) media are composed of complex materials, e.g. yeast extract, beef extract, and peptone (partially digested protein), therefore their chemical composition is poorly defined. On the other hand, these materials are rich in nutrients and vitamins.

3. *Function*

   - All-purpose media do not contain any special additives and they aim to support the growth of most bacteria.

   - Selective media enhance the growth of certain organisms while inhibit others due to the inclusion of particular substrate(s).

   - Differential media allow identification of microorganisms usually through their unique (and visible) physiological reactions. In the detection of common pathogens, most practical media are both selective and differential.

- Enrichment media contain specific growth factors that allow the growth of metabolically fastidious microorganisms. An enrichment culture is obtained with selected media and incubation conditions to isolate the microorganisms of interest.

### Sterilization of Culture Media

Although sterilization of culture media is best carried out in a steam autoclave at temperatures between 121–134°C, it has to be recognised that damage is caused to the medium by the heating process. Heat treatment of complex culture media which contain peptides, sugars, minerals and metals results in nutrient destruction, either by direct thermal degradation or by reaction between the medium components.

Toxic products caused by chemo-oxidation can also be formed during heat treatment. It is important, therefore, to optimise the heating process so that a medium is sterile after heating but minimal damage is caused to the ingredients of the medium. As a general rule it is accepted that short-duration, high-temperature processes are more lethal to organisms and less chemically damaging than are longer, lower temperature processes, e.g. 3 minutes at 134°C is preferable to 20 minutes at 115°C.

A general instruction for sterilizing culture media in volumes up to 1 litre at 121°C for 20 minutes is given on label of each commercially available media bottles. Autoclaves vary in performance, however, and thermocouple tests using different volumes of media should be carried out to determine the 'heat-up' and 'cool-down' times. It will be essential to do this when volumes of media greater than two litres are prepared. In order to avoid overheating large volume units of media, the 'heat-up' and 'cool-down' periods are normally integrated into the 121°C holding time.

### Sterilization Cycle

The sterilization cycle can be divided into four stages:

**Stage 1:** 20–121°C—chamber heat-up time.

The chamber heat-up time depends on the efficiency of the autoclave (air discharge/steam input) and the size of the load in the chamber. The time required for this stage is measured with a recording probe located in the air-discharge valve located in the base of the chamber.

**Stage 2:** 100–121°C—heat penetration time of the medium container.

The heat penetration time depends mainly on the volume of the individual containers, although the shape and the heat-transfer properties of the containers may affect this stage. The time required for the medium volume to reach 121°C is measured with thermocouples placed in the centre of the innermost container.

**Stage 3:** 121–121°C—holding time at the prescribed temperature.

The holding time at 121°C depends on (i) the number of organisms originally present in the medium, (ii) the fractional number of an organism presumed present after heating, e.g. N = 0.001 equivalent to one bottle in every 1000 bottles heated becoming contaminated, (iii) the thermal death rate constant of the presumed organism present at 121°C.

**Stage 4:** 121–80°C—cool-down time for the chamber to reach 80°C.

The cool-down time depends on the size of the load in the chamber and the heat loss rate from the autoclave. Water-sprays are used to accelerate cooling in commercial sterilizers but very careful control is required to avoid bottle fracture and the ingress of the cooling spray into the sterilized medium. The latter problem occurs when the vacuum formed in the head-space during cooling sucks contaminated cooling fluid up the thread of the cap and into the bottle.

Culture media autoclaves should be unlagged and of moderate chamber capacity only. Thermal locks on the doors should prevent them opening when the chamber temperature is above 80°C but even in these circumstances care should be taken to avoid sudden thermal shock when removing glass bottles of hot liquid from the autoclave. When screw-capped containers are placed in an autoclave, the caps should be a half-turn free to allow the escape of heated air. When removed from the autoclave, the containers should be allowed to cool down in a laminar airflow cabinet. Alternatively screw-capped containers may be sterilized in a jar which is covered by a piece of felt which effectively protects the containers from infection by airborne microorganisms. Caps are screwed down tightly after the contents have cooled to ambient temperature.

## Bibliography

1. Feazel, LM, Malhotra, A, Perencevich, EN, Kaboli, P, Diekema, DJ, and Schweizer, ML (2014). Effect of antibiotic stewardship programmes on Clostridium difficile incidence: a systematic review and meta-analysis. Journal of Antimicrobial Chemotherapy, 69(7), 1748–1754.
2. Phelan, K, and May, KM (2017). Mammalian cell tissue culture techniques. Current Protocols in Molecular Biology, A-3F.

**Aim:** To study the antimicrobial sensitivity of the given sample using Kirby-Bauer method.

**Principle:** Antibiotic sensitivity or antibiotic susceptibility is the susceptibility of bacteria to antibiotics. The Kirby-Bauer test, known as the disk-diffusion method, is the most widely used antibiotic susceptibility test. This method relies on the inhibition of bacterial growth measured under standard conditions. For this test, a culture medium, specifically the Müeller-Hinton agar, is uniformly and aseptically inoculated with the test organism and then filter paper discs, which are impregnated with a specific concentration of a particular antibiotic, are placed on the medium. The organism will grow on the agar plate while the antibiotic 'works' to inhibit the growth. If the organism is susceptible to a specific antibiotic, there will be no growth around the disc containing the antibiotic. Thus, a 'zone of inhibition' can be observed and measured to determine the susceptibility to an antibiotic for that particular organism. The size of this zone depends on how effective the antibiotic is at stopping the growth of the bacterium. A stronger antibiotic will create a larger zone, because a lower concentration of the antibiotic is enough to stop growth. The measurement is compared to the criteria set by the National Committee for Clinical Laboratory Studies (NCCLS). Based on the criteria, the organism can be classified as being resistant (R), intermediate (I), or susceptible (S).

### Requirements

*Chemicals:* Standard antimicrobial stock solution, test sample solution, agar media, distill water.

*Equipment:* Autoclave, incubator and water bath.

*Glasswares:* Conical flasks, beakers, pipettes, Petri dishes measuring cylinder and glass rod.

### Procedure

*I. Preparation of Müeller-Hinton Agar*

1. Müeller-Hinton agar should be prepared from a commercially available dehydrated base according to the manufacturer's instructions.
2. Immediately after autoclaving, allow it to cool in a 45–50°C water bath.
3. Pour the freshly prepared and cooled medium into glass or plastic, flat-bottomed Petri dishes on a level, horizontal surface to give a uniform

depth of approximately 4 mm. This corresponds to 60–70 mL of medium for plates with diameters of 150 mm and 25–30 mL for plates with a diameter of 100 mm.

4. The agar medium should be allowed to cool to room temperature and, unless the plate is used the same day, stored in a refrigerator (2–8°C).

5. Plates should be used within seven days after preparation unless adequate precautions, such as wrapping in plastic, have been taken to minimize drying of the agar.

6. A representative sample of each batch of plates should be examined for sterility by incubating at 30–35°C for 24 hours or longer.

## II. Preparation of Antibiotic Stock Solutions

1. Antibiotics may be received as powders or tablets. It is recommended to obtain pure antibiotics from commercial sources, and not use injectable solutions. Powders must be accurately weighed and dissolved in the appropriate diluents.

2. Standard strains of stock cultures should be used to evaluate the antibiotic stock solution. If satisfactory, the stock can be aliquoted in 5 mL volumes and frozen at –20°C or –60°C.

3. Stock solutions are prepared using the formula:

$$(1000/P) \times V \times C = W$$

where, P—potency of the antibiotic base

V—volume in mL required

C—final concentration of solution

W—weight of the antimicrobial to be dissolved in V

## III. Preparation of Dried Filter Paper Discs

1. Whatman filter paper no. 1 is used to prepare discs approximately 6 mm in diameter, which are placed in a Petri dish and sterilized in a hot air oven.

2. The loop used for delivering the antibiotics is made of 20 gauge wire and has a diameter of 2 mm. This delivers 0.005 mL of antibiotics to each disc.

## IV. Turbidity Standard for Inoculum Preparation

To standardize the inoculum density for a susceptibility test, a $BaSO_4$ turbidity standard, equivalent to a 0.5 McFarland standard or its optical equivalent (e.g. latex particle suspension), should be used.

## Preparation of BaSO$_4$ 0.5 McFarland standard:

1. A 0.5 mL aliquot of 0.048 mol/L BaCl$_2$ (1.175% w/v BaCl$_2$· 2H$_2$O) is added to 99.5 mL of 0.18 mol/L H$_2$SO$_4$ (1% v/v) with constant stirring to maintain a suspension.

2. The correct density of the turbidity standard should be verified by using a spectrophotometer with a 1 cm light path and matched cuvette to determine the absorbance. The absorbance at 625 nm should be 0.008–0.10 for the 0.5 McFarland standard.

3. The barium sulfate suspension should be transferred in 4–6 mL aliquots into screw-cap tubes of the same size as those used in growing or diluting the bacterial inoculum.

4. These tubes should be tightly sealed and stored in the dark at room temperature.

5. The barium sulfate turbidity standard should be vigorously agitated on a mechanical vortex mixer before each use and inspected for a uniformly turbid appearance. If large particles appear, the standard should be replaced.

6. The barium sulfate standards should be replaced or their densities verified monthly.

### V. Procedure for Performing the Disc Diffusion Test

**A. Inoculum preparation by growth method:** The growth method is performed as follows:

1. At least three to five well-isolated colonies of the same morphological type are selected from an agar plate culture. The top of each colony is touched with a loop, and the growth is transferred into a tube containing 4–5 mL of a suitable broth medium, such as tryptic soy broth.

2. The broth culture is incubated at 35°C until it achieves or exceeds the turbidity of the 0.5 McFarland standard (usually 2–6 hours).

3. The turbidity of the actively growing broth culture is adjusted with sterile saline or broth to obtain a turbidity optically comparable to that of the 0.5 McFarland standard. This results in a suspension containing approximately 1 to 2 × 10$^8$ CFU/mL (CFU, colony forming unit) for *E. coli* ATCC 25922 strain. To perform this step properly, either a photometric device can be used or, if done visually, adequate light is needed to visually compare the inoculum tube and the 0.5 McFarland standard against a card with a white background and contrasting black lines.

**B. Inoculum preparation by direct colony suspension method:**

1. As a convenient alternative to the growth method, the inoculum can be prepared by making a direct broth or saline suspension of isolated

colonies selected from a 18–24-hour agar plate (a nonselective medium, such as blood agar, should be used). The suspension is adjusted to match the 0.5 McFarland turbidity standard, using saline and a vortex mixer.

2. This approach is the recommended method for testing the fastidious organisms, Haemophilus spp., *N. gonorrhoeae*, and streptococci, and for testing staphylococci for potential methicillin or oxacillin resistance.

## VI. Inoculation of Test Plates

1. Optimally, within 15 minutes after adjusting the turbidity of the inoculum suspension, a sterile cotton swab is dipped into the adjusted suspension. The swab should be rotated several times and pressed firmly on the inside wall of the tube above the fluid level. This will remove excess inoculum from the swab.

2. The dried surface of a Müeller-Hinton agar plate is inoculated by streaking the swab over the entire sterile agar surface. This procedure is repeated by streaking two more times, rotating the plate approximately 60 each time to ensure an even distribution of inoculum. As a final step, the rim of the agar is swabbed.

3. The lid may be left ajar for 3–5 minutes, but no more than 15 minutes, to allow for any excess surface moisture to be absorbed before applying the drug impregnated disks.

*Note:* Extremes in inoculum density must be avoided. Never use undiluted overnight broth cultures or other unstandardized inocula for streaking plates.

## VI. Application of Discs to Inoculated Agar Plates

1. The predetermined battery of antimicrobial discs is dispensed onto the surface of the inoculated agar plate. Each disc must be pressed down to ensure complete contact with the agar surface. Whether the discs are placed individually or with a dispensing apparatus, they must be distributed evenly so that they are no closer than 24 mm from center to center. Ordinarily, no more than 12 discs should be placed on one 150 mm plate or more than 5 discs on a 100 mm plate. Because some of the drug diffuses almost instantaneously, a disc should not be relocated once it has come into contact with the agar surface. Instead, place a new disc in another location on the agar.

2. The plates are inverted and placed in an incubator set to 35°C within 15 minutes after the discs are applied (with the exception of Haemophilus spp. and streptococci).

## Observation

*Reading Plates and Interpreting Results*

1. After 16–18 hours of incubation, each plate is examined. If the plate was satisfactorily streaked, and the inoculum was correct, the resulting zones of inhibition will be uniformly circular and there will be a confluent lawn of growth (Fig. 6.1).

2. If individual colonies are apparent, the inoculum was too light and the test must be repeated. The diameters of the zones of complete inhibition (as judged by the unaided eye) are measured, including the diameter of the disc. Zones are measured to the nearest whole millimeter, using sliding calipers or a ruler, which is held on the back of the inverted Petri plate.

3. The Petri plate is held a few inches above a black, nonreflecting background and illuminated with reflected light. If blood was added to the agar base (as with streptococci), the zones are measured from the upper surface of the agar illuminated with reflected light, with the cover removed.

4. If the test organism is a Staphylococcus or Enterococcus spp., 24 hours of incubation are required for vancomycin and oxacillin, but other agents can be read at 16–18 hours. Transmitted light (plate held up to light) is used to examine the oxacillin and vancomycin zones for light growth of methicillin- or vancomycin-resistant colonies, respectively, within

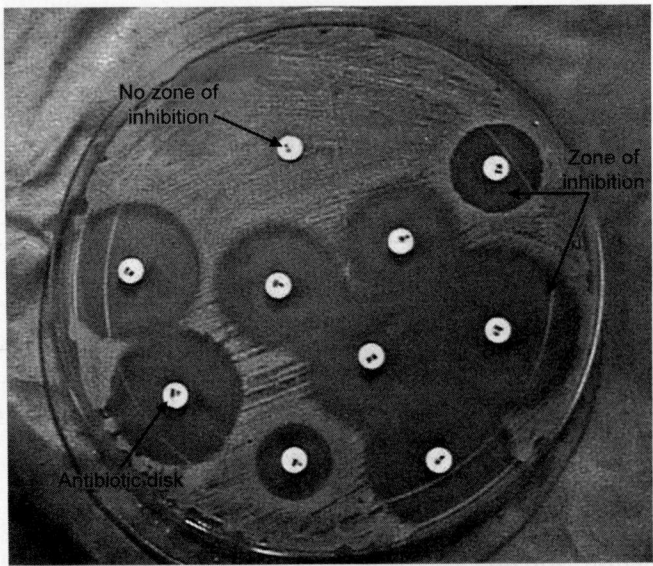

No zone of inhibition

Zone of inhibition

Antibiotic disk

**Fig. 6.1:** Antibiotic sensitivity test by Kirby-Bauer method

apparent zones of inhibition. Any discernable growth within zone of inhibition is indicative of methicillin or vancomycin resistance.

5. The zone margin should be taken as the area showing no obvious, visible growth that can be detected with the unaided eye. Faint growth of tiny colonies, which can be detected only with a magnifying lens at the edge of the zone of inhibited growth, is ignored. However, discrete colonies growing within a clear zone of inhibition should be subcultured, re-identified, and retested. Strains of Proteus spp. may swarm into areas of inhibited growth around certain antimicrobial agents. With Proteus spp., the thin veil of swarming growth in an otherwise obvious zone of inhibition should be ignored. When using blood-supplemented medium for testing streptococci, the zone of growth inhibition should be measured, not the zone of inhibition of hemolysis. With trimethoprim and the sulfonamides, antagonists in the medium may allow some slight growth; therefore, disregard slight growth (20% or less of the lawn of growth), and measure the more obvious margin to determine the zone diameter.

6. The diameter of the zone of inhibition is calibrated in millimeters and compared with the Interpretive Zone Standards published by the National Committee for Clinical Laboratory Standards. Results are reported as S (sensitive), I (intermediate), or R (resistant).

## Interpretation of Results

Measure the radius of the inhibition zone from the edge of the disc to the edge of the zone.

- Sensitive (S): Zone radius is wider than or equal to, or not more than 3 mm smaller than the control.
- Intermediate (I): Zone radius is >2 mm but smaller than the control by >3 mm.
- Resistant (R): No zone of inhibition or zone radius measures 2 mm or less.

## Bibliography

1. Lalitha, MK (2004). Manual on antimicrobial susceptibility testing. Performance standards for antimicrobial testing: Twelfth Informational Supplement, 56238, 454–456.

2. Wachino, JI, Kimura, K, Yamada, K, Jin, W, and Arakawa, Y (2014). Evaluation of Disk Potentiation Test Using Kirby-Bauer Disks Containing High-Dosage Fosfomycin and Glucose-6-Phosphate To Detect Production of Glutathione S-Transferase Responsible for Fosfomycin Resistance. Journal of Clinical Microbiology, 52(10), 3827–3828.

**Aim:** To study the antimicrobial sensitivity of the given sample using Stokes method.

**Principle:** Antibiotic sensitivity or antibiotic susceptibility is the susceptibility of bacteria to antibiotics. The Kirby-Bauer test, known as the disk-diffusion method, is the most widely used antibiotic susceptibility test. Stokes disc diffusion technique varies from Kirby-Bauer disc diffusion in the use of both control and test strain on a same plate. Stokes disc diffusion technique is not as highly standardized as the Kirby-Bauer technique and is used in laboratories particularly when the exact amount of antimicrobial in a disc cannot be guaranteed due to difficulties in obtaining discs and storing them correctly or when the other conditions required for the Kirby-Bauer technique cannot be met. The Stokes method allows each individual isolate to be compared with a sensitive control of the same or similar species which is subjected to the same technical conditions of medium, incubation time, atmosphere, temperature and disc content. As control and test organisms are adjacent on the same plate the difference between respective zone sizes can be measured directly.

### Requirements

*Chemicals:* Standard antimicrobial stock solution, test sample solution, agar media, distill water, trypsin soy broth and McFarland standard.

*Equipment:* Autoclave, incubator and water bath.

*Glasswares:* Conical flasks, beakers, pipettes, Petri dishes measuring cylinder and glass rod.

### Procedure

1. At least three to five well-isolated colonies of the same morphological type of both test and control strains are selected from an agar plate culture. The top of each colony is touched with a loop, and the growth is transferred into a tube containing 4–5 mL of a suitable broth medium, such as tryptic soy broth.
2. The broth culture is incubated at 37°C until it achieves or exceeds the turbidity of the 0.5 McFarland standard (usually 2–6 hours).
3. The turbidity of the actively growing broth culture is adjusted with sterile saline or broth to obtain a turbidity optically comparable to that of the 0.5 McFarland standard. This results in a suspension containing approximately 1 to $2 \times 10^8$ CFU/mL for *E. coli* ATCC 25922. To perform

this step properly, either a photometric device can be used, or if done visually, adequate light is needed to visually compare the inoculum tube and the 0.5 McFarland standard against a card with a white background and contrasting black lines.

4. Optimally, within 15 minutes after adjusting the turbidity of the inoculum and control strains suspension, sterile cotton swabs are dipped into each of the adjusted suspension. The swabs should be rotated several times and pressed firmly on the inside wall of the tube above the fluid level. This will remove excess inoculum from the swab.

5. A dried Müeller-Hinton agar plate is divided into 3 halves. The method of preparation of Müeller-Hinton agar plate is same as described in the previous experiments.

6. The dried surface of a Müeller-Hinton agar plate is inoculated by streaking the control strains evenly across the upper and lower thirds of the plate, and the test strains between the control, leaving a distance of not more than 5 mm on each side of the control strain.

7. Allow the inocula to dry for a few minutes with the lid.

8. Place antimicrobial discs in the gap between the test and control strain using a sterile forcep and press gently.

9. Within 30 minutes of applying the discs, incubate the plates aerobically at 35–37°C for 18–24 hours.

## Observation

### Reading Plates and Interpreting Results

1. After incubation, each plate is examined. If the plate was satisfactorily streaked, and the inoculum was correct, the resulting zones of inhibition will be uniformly circular and there will be a confluent lawn of growth (Fig. 6.2).

2. The diameter of the zone of inhibition is calibrated in millimeters and compared with the Interpretive Zone Standards published by the National Committee for Clinical Laboratory Standards. Results are reported as S (sensitive), I (intermediate), or R (resistant).

### Interpretation of Results

Measure the radius of the inhibition zone from the edge of the disc to the edge of the zone.

- **Sensitive (S):** Zone radius is wider than or equal to, or not more than 3 mm smaller than the control.

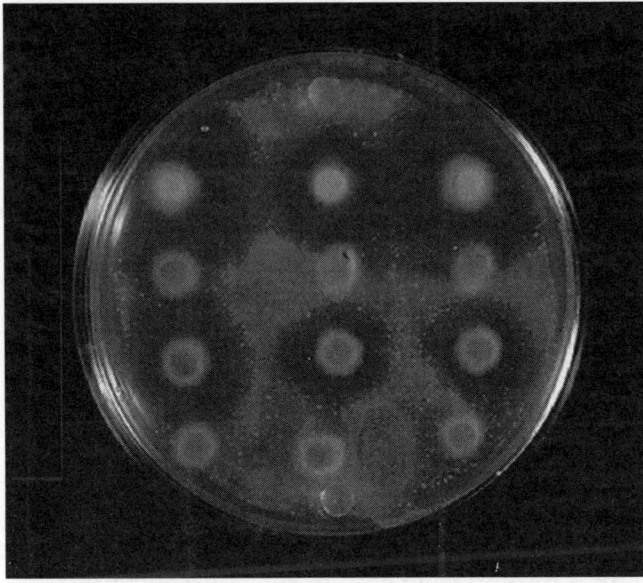

**Fig. 6.2:** Antibiotic sensitivity test by Stokes method
(Each row has separate concentration of sample)

- **Intermediate (I):** Zone radius is >2 mm but smaller than the control by >3 mm.
- **Resistant (R):** No zone of inhibition or zone radius measures 2 mm or less.

## Bibliography

1. Brown, DF, Wootton, M, and Howe, RA (2016). Antimicrobial susceptibility testing breakpoints and methods from BSAC to EUCAST. Journal of Antimicrobial Chemotherapy, 71(1), 3–5.
2. Lalitha, MK (2004). Manual on antimicrobial susceptibility testing. Performance standards for antimicrobial testing: Twelfth Informational Supplement, 56238, 454–456.
3. Piddock, LJ (1990). Techniques used for the determination of antimicrobial resistance and sensitivity in bacteria. Journal of Applied Bacteriology, 68(4), 307–318.

## EXPERIMENT 6.3

**Aim:** To determine the minimum inhibitory concentration (MIC) of the given sample using broth dilution method.

**Principle:** Minimum inhibitory concentration (MIC) is the lowest concentration of an antimicrobial that will inhibit the visible growth of a microorganism following overnight incubation, usually reported as mg/L. In other words, at which it has bacteriostatic activity. Diffusion tests widely used to determine the susceptibility of organisms isolated from clinical specimens have their limitations; when equivocal results are obtained or in prolonged serious infection, e.g. bacterial endocarditis, the quantitation of antibiotic action vis-à-vis the pathogen needs to be more precise. Also the terms 'Susceptible' and 'Resistant' can have a realistic interpretation. Thus, when in doubt, the way to a precise assessment is to determine the MIC of the antibiotic to the organisms concerned. Dilution susceptibility testing methods are used to determine the minimal concentration of antimicrobial to inhibit or kill the microorganism. This can be achieved by dilution of antimicrobial in either agar or broth media. Antimicrobials are tested in log 2 serial dilutions (twofold).

The broth dilution method is a simple procedure for testing a small number of isolates, even single isolate. It has the added advantage that the same tubes can be taken for minimum bacterial concentration (MBC) tests also.

### Requirements

*Chemicals:* Standard antimicrobial stock solution, test sample solution, agar media, overnight broth culture of test and control organisms, sterile distilled water 500 mL and suitable nutrient broth medium. Trimethoprim and sulphonamide testing requires thymidine free media or addition of 4% lysed horse blood to the media.

*Equipment:* Autoclave, incubator and water bath.

*Glasswares:* Conical flasks, beakers, measuring cylinder and glass rod, sterile graduated pipettes of 10 mL, 5 mL, 2 mL and 1 mL, sterile capped 7.5 × 1.3 cm tubes/small screw-capped bottles, Pasteur pipettes, a suitable rack to hold 22 tubes in two rows, i.e. 11 tubes in each row.

### Procedure

1. **Preparation of stock solution:** Stock solution can be prepared using the formula:
$$1000 \times V \times C = W \, P$$

where, P—potency given by the manufacturer in relation to the base

V—volume in mL required

C—final concentration of solution (multiples of 1000)

**Note:** The stock solutions are made in higher concentrations to maintain their keeping qualities and stored in suitable aliquots at –20°C. Once taken out, they should not be refrozen or reused.

2. Prepare stock dilutions of the antibiotic of concentrations 1000 and 100 µg/L as required from original stock solution (10,000 mg/L).

   *Calculations for the preparation of the original dilution*: This often presents problems to those unaccustomed to performing these tests. Calculate the total volume required for the first dilution. Two sets of dilution are being prepared (one for the test and one for the control), each in 2 mL volumes, i.e. a total of 4 mL for each concentration as 4 mL is required to make the second dilution, the total requirement is 8 mL. Now calculate the total amount of the antibiotic required for 8 mL.

3. Arrange two rows of 12 sterile 7.5 × 1.3 cm capped tubes in the rack.

4. In a sterile 30 mL (universal) screw-capped bottle, prepare 8 mL of broth containing the concentration of antibiotic required for the first tube in each row from the appropriate stock solution already made.

5. Mix the contents of the universal bottle using a pipette and transfer 2 mL to the first tube in each row. Using a fresh pipette, add 4 mL of broth to the remaining 4 mL in the universal bottle mix and transfer 2 mL to the second tube in each row.

6. Continue preparing dilutions in this way but where as many as 10 or more are required the series should be started again half the way down. Place 2 mL of antibiotic free broth to the last tube in each row.

7. Inoculate one row with one drop of an overnight broth culture of the test organism diluted approximately to 1 in 1000 in a suitable broth and the second row with the control organism of known sensitivity similarly diluted.

**Note:** The result of the test is significantly affected by the size of the inoculum. The test mixture should contain $10^6$ organism/mL. If the broth culture used has grown poorly, it may be necessary to use this undiluted.

8. Incubate tubes for 18 hours at 37°C. Inoculate a tube containing 2 mL broth with the organism and keep at +4°C in a refrigerator overnight to be used as standard for the determination of complete inhibition.

**Reading of result:** MIC is expressed as the lowest dilution, which inhibited growth judged by lack of turbidity in the tube.

Because very faint turbidity may be given by the inoculum itself, the inoculated tube kept in the refrigerator overnight may be used as the standard for the determination of complete inhibition.

Standard strain of known MIC value run with the test is used as the control to check the reagents and conditions.

## Bibliography

1. Lalitha, MK (2004). Manual on antimicrobial susceptibility testing. Performance standards for antimicrobial testing: Twelfth Informational Supplement, 56238, 454–456.
2. Wiegand, I, Hilpert, K, and Hancock, RE (2008). Agar and broth dilution methods to determine the minimal inhibitory concentration (MIC) of antimicrobial substances. Nature Protocols, 3(2), 163–175.

## EXPERIMENT 6.4

**Aim:** To determine the minimum inhibitory concentration (MIC) of the given sample using agar dilution method.

**Principle:** Minimum inhibitory concentration is the lowest concentration of an antimicrobial that will inhibit the visible growth of a microorganism following overnight incubation, usually reported as mg/L. In other words, at which it has bacteriostatic activity. Diffusion tests widely used to determine the susceptibility of organisms isolated from clinical specimens have their limitations; when equivocal results are obtained or in prolonged serious infection, e.g. bacterial endocarditis, the quantitation of antibiotic action vis-à-vis the pathogen needs to be more precise. Also the terms 'Susceptible' and 'Resistant' can have a realistic interpretation. Thus, when in doubt, the way to a precise assessment is to determine the MIC of the antibiotic to the organisms concerned. Dilution susceptibility testing methods are used to determine the minimal concentration of antimicrobial to inhibit or kill the microorganism. This can be achieved by dilution of antimicrobial in either agar or broth media. Antimicrobials are tested in log 2 serial dilutions (twofold).

Agar dilutions are most often prepared in Petri dishes and have advantage that it is possible to test several organisms on each plate. If only one organism is to be tested, e.g. *M. tuberculosis*, the dilutions can be prepared in agar slopes, but it will then be necessary to prepare a second identical set to be inoculated with the control organism. The dilutions are made in a small volume of water and added to agar which has been melted and cooled to not more than 60°C. Blood may be added and if 'chocolate agar' is required, the medium must be heated before the antibiotic is added.

### Requirements

*Chemicals:* Standard antimicrobial stock solution, test sample solution, agar media, overnight broth culture of test and control organisms, sterile distilled water 500 mL and suitable nutrient broth medium. Trimethoprim and sulphonamide testing requires thymidine free media or addition of 4% lysed horse blood to the media.

*Equipment:* Autoclave, incubator and water bath.

*Glasswares:* Conical flasks, beakers, measuring cylinder and glass rod Sterile graduated pipettes of 10 mL, 5 mL, 2 mL and 1 mL, sterile capped 7.5 × 1.3 cm tubes/small screw-capped bottles, Pasteur pipettes, a suitable rack to hold 22 tubes in two rows, i.e. 11 tubes in each row.

## Procedure

1. Label a sterile Petri dish on the base for each concentration required. Prepare the dilutions in water placing 1 mL of each in the appropriate dish. One mL water is added to a control plate.

2. Pipette 19 mL melted agar, cooled to 55°C to each plate and mix thoroughly. Adequate mixing is essential and if sufficient technical expertise is not available for the skilled manipulation, it is strongly recommended that the agar is first measured into stoppered tubes or universal containers and the drug dilution added to these and mixed by inversion before pouring into Petri dishes.

3. After the plates have set they should be well dried at 37°C with their lids tipped for 20–30 minutes in an incubator. They are then inoculated either with a multiple inoculator as spots or with a wire loop or a platinum loop calibrated to deliver 0.001 mL spread over a small area. In either case the culture should be diluted to contain $10^5$ to $10^6$ organisms per mL. With ordinary fast growing organisms, this can be obtained approximately by adding 5 µL of an overnight broth culture to 5 mL broth or peptone water.

**Reading of results:** The antibiotic concentration of the first plate showing 99% inhibition is taken as the MIC for the organism. A concentration dependent percentage growth inhibition graph can be plotted for the same.

## Bibliography

1. Lalitha, MK (2004). Manual on antimicrobial susceptibility testing. Performance standards for antimicrobial testing: Twelfth Informational Supplement, 56238, 454–456.

2. Wiegand, I, Hilpert, K, and Hancock, RE (2008). Agar and broth dilution methods to determine the minimal inhibitory concentration (MIC) of antimicrobial substances. Nature Protocols, 3(2), 163–175.

## EXPERIMENT 6.5

**Aim:** To determine the minimum bactericidal concentration (MBC) of the given sample using broth dilution test.

**Principle:** The minimum bactericidal concentration is the concentration that results in microbial death (in other words, the concentration at which it is bactericidal). The broth dilution method is a simple procedure for testing a small number of isolates, even single isolate. It has the added advantage that the same tubes can be taken for MBC tests also.

### Requirements

*Chemicals:* Standard antimicrobial stock solution, test sample solution, agar media, overnight broth culture of test and control organisms, sterile distilled water 500 mL and suitable nutrient broth medium. Trimethoprim and sulphonamide testing requires thymidine free media or addition of 4% lysed horse blood to the media.

*Equipment:* Autoclave, incubator and water bath.

*Glasswares:* Conical flasks, beakers, measuring cylinder and glass rod sterile graduated pipettes of 10 mL, 5 mL, 2 mL and 1 mL sterile capped 7.5 × 1.3 cm tubes/small screw-capped bottles, Pasteur pipettes, a suitable rack to hold 22 tubes in two rows, i.e. 11 tubes in each row.

### Procedure

1. Dilutions and inoculations are prepared in the same manner as described for the determination of MIC. The control tube containing no antibiotic is immediately subcultured (before incubation) by spreading a loopful evenly over a quarter of the plate on a medium suitable for the growth of the test organism and incubated at 37°C overnight.

2. The tubes are also incubated overnight at 37°C. Read the MIC of the control organism to check that the drug concentrations are correct.

*Note:* The lowest concentration inhibiting growth of the organisms and record this as the MIC.

3. Subculture all tubes not showing visible growth in the same manner as the control tube described above and incubate at 37°C overnight. Compare the amount of growth from the control tube before incubation, which represents the original inoculum.

4. The test must include a second set of the same dilutions inoculated with an organism of known sensitivity. These tubes are not subcultured; the purpose of the control is to confirm by its MIC that the drug level is correct, whether or not this organism is killed is immaterial.

## Reading of Result

These subcultures may show:

- Similar number of colonies indicating bacteriostasis only.
- A reduced number of colonies indicating a partial or slow bactericidal activity.
- No growth if the whole inoculum has been killed.
- The highest dilution showing at least 99% inhibition is taken as MBC.

**Alternate method:** Micro-broth dilution test.

This test uses double-strength Müeller-Hinton broth (MHB), 4× strength antibiotic solutions prepared as serial twofold dilutions and the test organism at a concentration of $2 \times 10^6$/mL. In a 96-well plate, 100 L of double-strength MHB, 50 L each of the antibiotic dilutions and the organism suspension are mixed and incubated at 35°C for 18–24 hours. The lowest concentration showing inhibition of growth will be considered the MIC of the organism.

**Reading of result:** MIC is expressed as the highest dilution which inhibited growth judged by lack of turbidity in the tube. Because very faint turbidity may be given by the inoculum itself the inoculated tube kept in the refrigerator overnight may be used as the standard for the determination of complete inhibition. Standard strain of known MIC, run with the test is used as the control to check the reagents and conditions.

## Bibliography

1. Lalitha, MK (2004). Manual on antimicrobial susceptibility testing. Performance standards for antimicrobial testing: Twelfth Informational Supplement, 56238, 454–456.
2. Owuama, CI (2017). Determination of minimum inhibitory concentration (MIC) and minimum bactericidal concentration (MBC) using a novel dilution tube method. African Journal of Microbiology Research, 11(23), 977–980.

## EXPERIMENT 6.6

**Aim:** To study the *in vitro* β-lactamase inhibitory potential of the given sample using β-lactamase inhibition assay.

**Principle:** The enzyme β-lactamase is produced by bacteria as a part of a resistance mechanism against β-lactam-containing antibiotics. A large number of β-lactamases have already been identified. β-Lactamases (often called penicillinases, cephalosporinases or carbapenemases, depending on substrate specificity) are plasmid or chromosomally encoded bacterial enzymes which inactivate β-lactam antibiotics. The enzyme efficiently hydrolyzes the amide bond of the β-lactam moiety, thereby yielding products devoid of antibiotic activity.

The clinical importance of β-lactamase inhibitors is reflected from the fact that most commonly used antimicrobial agents are β-lactam-containing antibiotics like penicillins, cephalosporins, carbapenems and monobactams. Because of the safety profiles and proven clinical efficacy, these antibiotics are extensively used for the treatment of many infectious diseases. The search for new β-lactamase inhibitors therefore has a tremendous clinical and commercial potential.

The measurement of the amount of antibiotics hydrolyzed per unit time can be followed spectrophotometrically by the increase in the absorbance at 495 nm due to hydrolysis of the highly conjugated cephalosporin. Although other penicillins or cephalosporins may be used as substrates in this assay, nitrocefin has the widest spectrum of susceptibility and sensitivity among the commercialy available β-lactam containing antibiotics (for other substrates the UV wavelength range depends upon the nature of the substrate).

### Requirements

*Chemicals:* Test sample, hyaluronidase enzyme, phosphate buffer (pH 7), calcium chloride ($CaCl_2$), potassium hyaluronate, potassium tetraborate, sodium hydroxide (NaOH) and *p*-dimethylaminobenzaldehyde (*p*-DMAB).

*Equipment:* UV-visible spectrophotometer.

*Glasswares:* Test tubes, micropipettes, measuring cylinder and glass rod.

### Procedure

1. Preincubate the test sample with the enzyme for 5–10 minutes.
2. To prepare enzyme solution dissolve it in 0.5 mL dimethylsulfoxide (DMSO). Add phosphate buffer (100 mmol/L, pH 7.0) to give a final

volume of 50 mL. Store in dark bottle at 4°C (if protected from light this solution maintains greater than 90% stability after storage for 2 weeks). β-lactamase from *Staphylococcus aureus* generally sticks on glass surfaces, therefore, disposable cuvettes should be used for assays of enzymes or glass cuvettes should be rinsed properly with ethanol before adding new samples to prevent carryover of the active enzyme.

3. Start reaction by adding 1.0 mL of substrate solution. Prepare substrate solution by dissolving 5.0 ± 0.2 mg nitrocefin into a 50 mL volumetric flask.

4. Although other penicillins or cephalosporins may be used as substrates in this assay, nitrocefin has the widest spectrum of susceptibility and sensitivity among the commercialy available lactam containing antibiotics (for other substrates the UV wavelength range depends upon the nature of the substrate).

5. Mix well using a plastic mixing spoon.

6. Read absorbance at 495 nm, and start stopwatch. Repeat readings exactly every 15 seconds or monitor on a recorder.

## Observation

| S. no. | Absorbance of control | Absorbance of test | Absorbance of standard |
|--------|----------------------|--------------------|------------------------|
| 1. | | | |
| 2. | | | |
| 3. | | | |

**Calculation:** The percentage inhibition of enzyme is calculated as follows:

$$\% \text{ inhibition of } \beta\text{-lactamase} = \frac{(\text{Abs control} - \text{Abs sample})}{\text{Abs control}} \times 100$$

where,  Abs control—absorbance of control

Abs sample—absorbance of sample

## Bibliography

1. Chantemesse, B, Betelli, L, Solanas, S, Vienney, F, Bollache, L, Hartmann, A, and Rochelet, M (2017). A nitrocefin-based amperometric assay for the rapid quantification of extended-spectrum β-lactamase-producing *Escherichia coli* in wastewaters. Water Research, 109, 375–381.

2. Vinutha, B, Prashanth, D, Salma, K, Sreeja, SL, Pratiti, D, Padmaja, R, and Deepak, M (2007). Screening of selected Indian medicinal plants for acetylcholinesterase inhibitory activity. Journal of Ethnopharmacology, 109(2), 359–363.

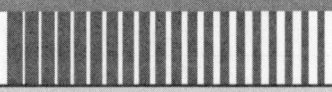

# CHAPTER 7

# *In vitro* Assay for Tropical Disease

WHO defines tropical diseases as diseases that occur solely, or principally, in the tropics. In practice, the term is often taken to refer to infectious diseases that thrive in hot, humid conditions, such as malaria, leishmaniasis, schistosomiasis, onchocerciasis, lymphatic filariasis, Chagas disease, African trypanosomiasis, and dengue. Neglected tropical diseases (NTDs) are a major public health problem globally as well as in India. The World Health Organization recognizes seventeen (17) major parasitic and related infections as the neglected tropical diseases out of which leishmaniasis and malaria are most prominent ones in India.

## LEISHMANIASIS

Leishmaniasis is caused by a protozoan parasite from over 20 Leishmania species and is transmitted to humans by the bite of infected female phlebotomine sandflies. Over 90 sandfly species are known to transmit Leishmania parasites. There are three main forms of the disease:

- **Visceral leishmaniasis (VL),** also known as kala-azar is fatal if left untreated in over 95% of cases. It is characterized by irregular bouts of fever, weight loss, enlargement of the spleen and liver, and anemia. It is highly endemic in the Indian subcontinent and in East Africa. An estimated 50,000–90,000 new cases of VL occur worldwide each year. In 2015, more than 90% of new cases reported to WHO occurred in 7 countries—Brazil, Ethiopia, India, Kenya, Somalia, South Sudan and Sudan. The kala-azar elimination programmes in South-East Asia are making sustained progress towards elimination, and cases are declining in the three major endemic countries—Bangladesh, India, and Nepal.
- **Cutaneous leishmaniasis (CL)** is the most common form of leishmaniasis and causes skin lesions, mainly ulcers, on exposed parts of the body,

leaving life-long scars and serious disability. About 95% of CL cases occur in the Americas, the Mediterranean basin, the Middle East and Central Asia. Over two-thirds of new CL cases are predominantly prevalent in 6 countries—Afghanistan, Algeria, Brazil, Colombia, Iran (Islamic Republic of) and the Syrian Arab Republic. An estimated 0.6–1 million new cases occur worldwide annually.

- **Mucocutaneous leishmaniasis** leads to partial or total destruction of mucous membranes of the nose, mouth and throat. Over 90% of mucocutaneous leishmaniasis cases occur in Bolivia, Brazil, Ethiopia, and Peru.

Leishmania parasites are transmitted through the bites of infected female phlebotomine sandflies. The epidemiology of leishmaniasis depends on the characteristics of the parasite species, the local ecological characteristics of the transmission sites, current and past exposure of the human population to the parasite, and human behavior. Some 70 animal species, including humans, have been found as natural reservoir hosts of Leishmania parasites.

## MALARIA

According to the latest world malaria report, released in November 2017, there were 216 million cases of malaria in 2016, up from 211 million cases in 2015. The estimated number of deaths due to malaria stood at approximately 445,000 in 2016, a similar number to the previous year (446000). The disease is caused by Plasmodium parasites. The parasites are spread in humans through the bites of infected female Anopheles mosquitoes, called 'malaria vectors.' There are five parasite species that cause malaria in humans, and two of these species—*P. falciparum* and *P. vivax* pose the greatest threat.

Malaria is an acute febrile illness. In a nonimmune individual, symptoms usually appear 10–15 days after the infective mosquito bite. The first symptoms—fever, headache, and chills—may be mild and difficult to recognize as malaria. If not treated within 24 hours, *P. falciparum* malaria can progress to severe illness, often leading to death.

Children with severe malaria frequently develop one or more of the following symptoms—severe anemia, respiratory distress in relation to metabolic acidosis, or cerebral malaria. In adults, multiorgan involvement is also frequent. In malaria endemic areas, people may develop partial immunity, allowing asymptomatic infections to occur.

In order to accurately define the antimalarial potency of any new lead molecule, it is necessary to be familiar with the varying stages of malaria as exhibited both in human and animal species. Figure 7.1 explains the life cycle of the malarial parasite also given below is a brief description of the different stages of malaria as exhibited in both humans and animal models used for preclinical assays.

**Human malaria:** In humans malarial parasites are preferentially harvested from either in exoerythrocytic stage or erythrocytic stage.

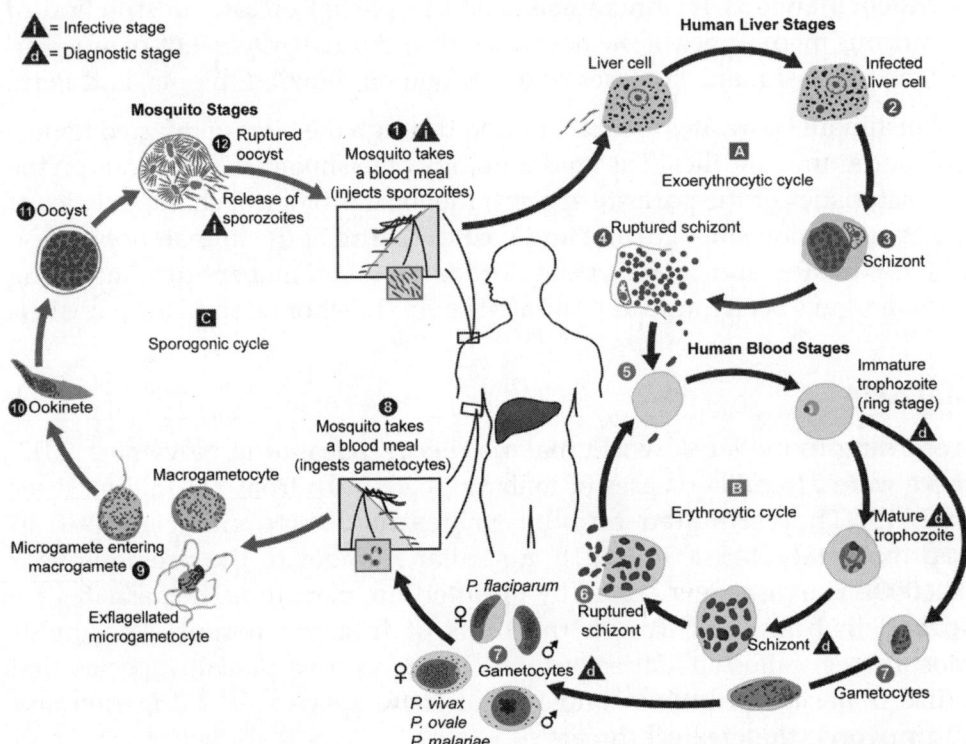

**Fig. 7.1:** Life cycle of malarial parasite both in host and vector

The malaria parasite life cycle involves two hosts. During a blood meal, a malaria-infected female Anopheles mosquito inoculates sporozoites into the human host (1), sporozoites infect liver cells (2) and mature into schizonts, which rupture and release merozoites (4). Of note, in *P. vivax* and *P. ovale* a dormant stage (hypnozoites) can persist in the liver and cause relapses by invading the bloodstream weeks, or even years later.) After this initial replication in the liver (exoerythrocytic schizogony) (A), the parasites undergo asexual multiplication in the erythrocytes (erythrocytic schizogony) (B). Merozoites infect red blood cells (5). The ring stage trophozoites mature into schizonts, which rupture releasing merozoites (5). Some parasites differentiate into sexual erythrocytic stages (gametocytes) (7). Blood stage parasites are responsible for the clinical manifestations of the disease. The gametocytes, male (microgametocytes) and female (macrogametocytes), are ingested by an Anopheles mosquito during a blood meal (8). The parasites' multiplication in the mosquito is known as the sporogonic cycle (C). While in the mosquito's stomach, the microgametes penetrate the macrogametes generating zygotes (9). The zygotes in turn become motile and elongated (ookinetes) (10) which invade the midgut wall of the mosquito where they develop into oocysts (11). The oocysts grow, rupture, and release sporozoites (12), which make their way to the mosquito's salivary glands. Inoculation of the sporozoites (1) into a new human host perpetuates the malaria life cycle.

## Exoerythrocytic Stages

When the Plasmodium parasite is first introduced into the bloodstream of its vertebrate host by the mosquito vector, the sporozoite stage parasite invades hepatic cells. In the case of *P. falciparum*, the parasite is probably taken up first by the Kupffer cells of the liver sinusoids in their passage to liver hepatocytes. Invading sporozoites developed into schizonts in host cells, with modest yields of about 650 schizonts/35 mm diameter culture dish. Addition of human erythrocytes to infected hepatocyte cultures resulted in appearance of ring-stage organisms in the blood cells, indicating production of merozoites infective for erythrocytes. The pattern of relapse that occurs with the human malarias caused by *P. vivax* and *P. ovale* is associated with the presence of dormant parasites termed hypnozoites that survive in the liver parenchymal cells of the host.

## Erythrocytic Stages

The greatest amounts of effort and time have been invested in cultivation of the erythrocytic stages in the Plasmodium life cycle, this being the stage most often associated with the pathogenesis of malaria and a major target for vaccine development. A significant accomplishment in this area is defining *in vitro* conditions for continuous cultivation of *P. falciparum*, the most important and deadly of the human malarial parasites. This was accomplished by Trager and Jensen using HEPES buffered Roswell Park Memorial Institute (RPMI) medium 1640, a tissue culture medium developed for *in vitro* cultivation of leukocytes, supplemented with human serum, erythrocytes, and sodium bicarbonate. Parasites can be cultured initially in Petri plates placed in a candle jar that provided an atmosphere of 3% $CO_2$ and 17% $O_2$ or in vials that allowed for continuous flow of medium into culture vessels with an atmosphere of 7% $CO_2$, 1% $O_2$ and 92% $N_2$. Currently $CO_2$ incubators are used for purpose of incubation.

### Serum as Medium Supplement

The growth system functions best with 10–15% human serum as a supplement. For reasons that include cost, reproducibility, and possible presence of inhibitory immune factors and antimalarial drugs, there is interest in substituting other types of mammalian sera (bovine, monkey, horse, goat, sheep, rabbit, or swine) for human serum or even developing a serum-free medium for parasite cultivation. In comparing horse, swine, and lamb sera, horse serum was superior to the others but not as good as human serum.

*Serum Replacements*

Freshly prepared human high-density lipoprotein fraction (concentration range of 0.25–0.50 mg/mL) can be used to support growth of *P. falciparum*. Other lipoprotein fractions, low- and very-low-density lipoproteins, produced little or no growth. Growth-promoting factor GF 21 (containing an ammonium sulfate fraction of adult bovine serum plus insulin, transferrin, and sodium selenite) was used with Daigo's T basal medium for serum-free growth of *P. falciparum*. Roswell Park Memorial Institute (RPMI) medium 1640 is supplemented with adenosine, unsaturated C18 fatty acids, and fatty acid-free bovine serum albumin for serum-free growth, but growth rates of parasites were lower than those in plasma-containing medium.

*Commercial Serum Replacements*

Examples of some commercially available media are as follows:

- Nutridoma-SR (4%) helps to support the growth of several strains of *P. falciparum* from different global locations, with a resulting parasitaemia of about 10% within 3–4 days. For better results using a lower concentration of nutridoma-SR (1%) combined can be combined with albumax I (0.5%), a purified serum albumin preparation.

- Albumax can be used for cultivation of *P. falciparum*, with parasitaemias reaching as high as 85% after 7 days with continuously passaged plasmodia. It is, however, necessary to add hypoxanthine to the growth medium in order to obtain adequate levels of parasitaemia.

- Plasma, without prior heat treatment, has been used for large scale growth of *P. falciparum*; clotting can be avoided by use of plastic culture vessels or siliconized glassware.

## Basal Medium

The tissue culture medium RPMI 1640 remains the medium of choice, not only for *P. falciparum* but also for most other Plasmodium spp. that have been cultured *in vitro*. Better consistency for parasite growth is obtained by preparing the medium from a powdered preparation rather than using the liquid form available from most suppliers. The medium is supplemented with hypoxanthine as a purine source. RPMI 1640 has been supplemented with additional glucose, hypoxanthine, and reduced glutathione to improve parasite yield.

*Role of the Erythrocyte in the Culture System*

Red blood cells are essential for development of the parasite, providing not only a location for asexual reproduction but also a source of nutrients for the parasite over and above that present in supplemented RPMI 1640. *In vivo* or *in vitro*, the parasite enters into the erythrocyte across the membrane and is enclosed in a vacuole, the parasitophorous vacuole, that forms in part from the membrane of the red blood cell. The malaria parasite takes in nutrients and develops into a multinucleate schizont which undergoes fission to produce a characteristic number of merozoites which, upon rupture of the parasitized blood cell, invade other blood cells and repeat the growth cycle.

Human blood cells of all groups are suitable for growth of *P. falciparum*. Type O cells are useful because of their compatibility with serum or plasma of all other blood groups. Type AB serum is compatible with any type of red blood cells. Citrated red blood cells may be stored for up to 5 weeks, at which time they become too fragile to use in cultures. Citrated red blood cells are washed and prepared as a 50% erythrocyte suspension which remains usable for 4 days at 4°C. Saline-adenine-glucose stored blood cells were found to improve parasite yield.

## Culture Systems

Plate cultures are prepared with a 5% hematocrit and about 1% parasitaemia. The lower the initial parasitaemia is, the greater the increase in numbers of parasites that will occur during *in vitro* growth is. Monitoring of parasitaemia is accomplished by preparing blood films, staining with Giemsa stain following methanol fixation, and counting infected red blood cells microscopically. While the simplest system for cultivation of parasites uses petri or Linbro plates in a candle jar, this system is labor-intensive, requiring constant attention and daily changes of medium in order to maintain parasite growth. In this static system infected erythrocytes settle out to form a layer, producing microenvironments high in lactic acid in the region of the proliferating parasites. This may lead to conditions unfavorable for schizont development and penetration of merozoites into uninfected erythrocytes. Lactic acid production taxes the buffering capacity of the medium and leads to a drop in pH, which is detrimental to the growth of Plasmodium. Optimal parasite yields occurred with an extracellular pH of 7.2–7.45 and a lactate concentration below 12 mM; higher lactate concentrations were postulated to cause negative feedback of glycolysis. Glucose diffusion into the cell layer also becomes limiting.

Several devices to semiautomate cultivation of plasmodia have been described previously. These devices allow for continuous flow of medium through growth vessels, with a controlled gas phase of 2–5% $CO_2$, 3–18% $O_2$, and the remainder being $N_2$. Semiautomated devices reduce the amount of time spent on maintenance of stock cultures of the parasite. Although the malarial parasite is found in red blood cells, it is microaerophilic in its oxygen preference.

### Induction of Synchrony In vitro

In its human host, *P. falciparum* exhibits a synchrony of about 48-hour duration.

Blood sampled at any one time from an infected host will reveal a parasite population at the same stage in its developmental cycle, i.e. mostly ring stages or mostly schizonts, etc. This synchrony is in part a response to the circadian rhythmicity of the host's body. Synchrony can be artificially imposed *in vitro* upon developing malaria parasites by one of several methods. Most popular is the use of sorbitol or mannitol treatment of infected erythrocytes. Infected cells are treated with 5% sorbitol, which causes lysis of erythrocytes containing late stages and preferentially selects for red blood cells with early ring stages. The effect is not osmotic, but has to do with the permeability of infected cells and the sensitivity of the parasites to sorbitol. Treatment can be repeated at 34 hours to further select for young stages and improve on the synchrony.

Most strains of *P. falciparum* produce knobs over the surface of the host erythrocyte when the parasite reaches the late trophozoite to schizont stage. Such red cells do not form rouleaux in the plasma gel, as do uninfected red cells or those containing ring-stage organisms. As a result, the cells with late-stage parasites remain in suspension while the uninfected ones and those with rings settle out. If the late-stage parasites are then mixed with fresh red cells and put under culture conditions, merozoites formed by them invade new cells. If one allows invasion to go on for 3 hours and then treats the cells with sorbitol to kill all late-stage parasites, one gets a population of rings just 0–3 hours old. Such a tightly synchronized culture will remain quite synchronous through about three cycles.

Shifting cultures of *P. falciparum* from 37 to 28°C has been used to delay the asexual cycle for 12–16 hours. Feeder cells either mouse peritoneal macrophages or the flagellated protozoon. *Crithidia fasciculate* can be used for establishment of *P. falciparum in vitro* with a success rate better than 80%. It is worth noting that cultured *P. falciparum* retains its infectivity and immunogenicity. In a laboratory accident, a puncture wound resulted in inoculation of cultured parasites leading to human infection with a strain that had been maintained *in vitro* for approximately 4 years (Table 7.1 for *in vitro* cultivation of human Plasmodium species).

### Plasmodium Spp. other than P. falciparum

Although the *in vitro* system has worked well for *P. falciparum*, *P. vivax* has not been amenable to cultivation using the same methods. SCMI 612

**Table 7.1:** *In vitro* cultivation of stages of human Plasmodium spp.[a]

| Stage | Species | Basal medium[a] | Additional factors |
|---|---|---|---|
| Exoerythrocytic | *P. falciparum* | MEM<br>RPMI 1640-MEM | Hepatoma cells |
| | *P. malariae* | MEM | Chimpanzee primary hepatocytes |
| | *P. ovale* | Arginine-free Ham's medium | Human and rat hepatocytes |
| | *P. vivax* | MEM | Hepatoma cells |
| Erythrocytic | *P. falciparum* | RPMI 1640<br>Semidefined medium | |
| | | RPMI 1640 | Cell-free system with Matrigel |
| | | Malaria culture medium | Feeder cells<br>(*C. fasciculata*) |
| | *P. malariae* | RPMI 1640 | Glutamine, hypoxanthine |
| | *P. vivax* | SCMI 612 | Elevated glucose |
| | | RPMI 1640 | Reticulocytes |
| | | McCoy's 5A | Reticulocytes |
| Gametocyte | *P. falciparum* | RPMI 1640 | Hypoxanthine |
| | | RPMI 1640 | Hormonal stimulation (insulin, etc.) |
| Sporogonic | *P. falciparum* | RPMI 1640 | Drosophila cells and Matrigel |

[a]Summary of the different media used for cultivation of the several species of the malaria parasite and their different stages.

medium can be used for schizogonic stages of *P. vivax* and found that this medium worked better than either RPMI 1640 or Weymouth media. They reported that a higher glucose level (3 mg/mL) was needed for *P. vivax* than for *P. falciparum*. Unlike *P. falciparum*, which develops in erythrocytes, *P. vivax* invades developing erythrocytes, the reticulocytes. Thus, in order to maintain this species *in vitro*, a large supply of reticulocytes is needed for development. RPMI 1640 medium with an enriched reticulocyte fraction from owl monkeys (Aotus spp.) can be used for cultivating *P. vivax*, noting that *P. vivax* preferentially infects these immature erythrocytes. Not only are reticulocytes necessary for parasite development, but agitation of the culture medium is also needed to establish contact between parasite and host cell.

A variety of supplements including hypoxanthine, ascorbic acid, choline, biotin, $B_{12}$, and $MgCl_2$ had little or no effect on growth and schizogony. Methyl cellulose (0.1%) is added to reduce breakage of erythrocyte membranes. Other supplements included glucose, spermidine, and antioxidants. *In vitro* cultivation of *P. vivax* for eight growth cycles can be achieved by the use of enriched populations of reticulocytes from humans with hemochromatosis. Using McCoy's 5A medium supplemented with glutamine and 20% human serum, culture of parasite initially in a candle jar until schizogonic stages can be obtained. The reticulocytes are then added and the culture is transferred to a shaker, which promoted contact between parasites and host cells. 85% ring-stage organisms are obtained after about 12 hours under these conditions. Gametocytes did not develop, although the parasites remained infective for owl monkeys.

### Cell-free Development of Erythrocytic Stages

While *in vitro* growth of plasmodia is a significant accomplishment in its own right, growth of the parasites under a completely cell-free or axenic condition would allow examination of the parasites' nutritional needs, biochemical and molecular properties, and sensitivity to antimicrobial agents, in the absence of those of the host erythrocyte. Towards this end, *P. falciparum* merozoites can be cultured to ring and trophic stages in HEPES buffered RPMI 1640 in which NaCl can be replaced by KCl, in the presence of a serum-supplemented, frozen-thawed 33% erythrocyte extract; dipotassium ATP (1.6 mM); and pyruvate (3.6 mM). Ultrastructural evidence indicate absence of the parasitophorous membrane in these extracellular forms, yet development occurred, suggesting that factors present in the erythrocyte but not necessarily the intracytoplasmic location of the parasite were needed for development. In a later study, it was found that sonicated erythrocyte preparations (about 50% erythrocyte extract), with ATP (2 mM) and pyruvate (5 mM) added, supported better development of extracellular *P. falciparum* than did frozen-thawed preparations, with about 30% of the merozoites developing to later stages. These extracellular forms react to the same monoclonal antibodies that the intracellular forms respond to, suggesting a similar pattern of molecular differentiation.

### Biphasic Cultivation System

Further refinement of the technique for axenic cultivation involved the use of a biphasic system with merozoites embedded in a Matrigel substrate in a well containing a fluid medium overlay. Coenzyme A, added as a supplement to the basic medium (0.15 mM), may enhance formation of later stages in the life cycle, though its role is not clear. The fluid medium could be changed with minimal disturbance to the parasites developing within the Matrigel layer. Ring-stage parasites developing within Matrigel attained larger sizes and showed motility, though only about 1% of the merozoites inoculated completed the asexual cycle *in vitro*. Gametocytes were observed in cultures after 36–44 hours of incubation.

Contact between parasite and spectrin in the erythrocyte sonicate may be an important factor for development. The yields of schizonts forming extracellularly can be increased by addition of erythrocyte ghosts obtained by osmotic lysis, to double the amount of membrane present. These results support the critical role of the erythrocyte membrane in the development of the malarial parasite. The role of Matrigel, a preparation of solubilized tissue basement membrane, may be simply to provide the parasite with a substrate that approximates the cytoplasmic matrix in which the merozoites begin to develop. Matrigel has also been an important factor in cultivation of the mosquito stages of the *P. falciparum* life cycle (*see* below).

## Gametocytogenesis

Gametocytes are the precursors of the macrogamete (female gamete) and the sperm cell which fuse to form a motile, banana-shaped zygote, the ookinete, in the wall of the gut of the mosquito. *In vivo*, gametocyte development occurs within erythrocytes in the peripheral circulatory system of the vertebrate host. These stages are picked up by the blood-sucking mosquito, in which they complete the sexual cycle of the malaria parasite. *In vitro*, variation exists among different strains of *P. falciparum* with respect to gametocyte formation, and even among different clones from the same strain of parasite.

## Induction of Gamete Formation

Gametocyte formation in cultures can be enhanced by changing the growth medium without providing fresh erythrocytes. Culture conditions also affect gametocytogenesis of *P. falciparum*. Strains recently isolated are more likely to form gametocytes than are strains that have been in culture over long periods of time. Hypoxanthine is necessary for induction and maturation of gametocytes forming in cultures of *P. falciparum*; without hypoxanthine, mosquitoes feeding on gametocyte-containing cultures would not develop oocyst infections. Some ammonium compounds (ammonium carbonate or ammonium bicarbonate, but not ammonium chloride or ammonium acetate) with or without concanavalin A trigger gametocyte formation on the third day following treatment. Evidence that signal transduction is involved in gametocytogenesis comes from several studies in which secondary messengers, or compounds affecting them, have been shown to enhance gametocyte formation. Also, cyclic AMP (cAMP) and dibutyryl cAMP (1 mM) increased gamete formation in *P. falciparum*. Phorbol compounds (phorbol 12-myristate-13-acetate and phorbol dibutyrate) and a phosphodiesterase inhibitor (8-bromo cAMP) can be employed to promote gametocyte production by 50% or more in cultured *P. falciparum*.

### Problems with Induction

Unlike the asexual division cycle that occurs within erythrocytes over a 48-h period, maturation of gametocytes of *P. falciparum* requires about 2 weeks. Nutrients present within the infected erythrocyte would be exhausted by the developing parasite over this prolonged time period and may be a factor in the difficulty of inducing gametocyte formation *in vitro*. Immature erythrocytes (reticulocytes) supported better gametocyte formation than did mature erythrocytes. Other factors affecting gametocyte formation may include variations in nutrients present in serum supplements of growth medium, absence of essential activating factors in RPMI 1640, and selection of nongametocyte-forming populations under *in vitro* conditions.

### Sporogonic Stages

The mosquito acquires gametocytes from the blood of a vertebrate. Development of the gametocytes into male and female gametes is initiated within the gut of the mosquito. The fused gametes form an ookinete, which develops into the oocyst in the hemocoel of the insect. Sporozoites develop within the oocyst and migrate to the salivary glands of the mosquito, to be injected into the next vertebrate host that the insect bites. A different set of growth conditions is needed for the successful cultivation of these stages of the *P. falciparum* life cycle. Warburg and Schneider successfully produced sporozoites of *P. falciparum* in a complex culture of *Drosophila melanogaster* cells and a Matrigel substrate, to which ookinetes adhered. Development of sporozoites took 12–16 days. Wheat germ agglutinin was used to enhance transformation of zygotes into retorts and ookinetes, by providing a modifying environment approximating conditions in the mosquito stomach for development of the sexual stages. Table 7.2 presents a summary of the stages of human malarial parasites and the types of media, and supplements that have been used in the cultivation.

## NONHUMAN MALARIA

Malarial parasites develop in the blood of many different vertebrates. In this section, attention will focus on *in vitro* cultured malarial parasites infecting simian, avian, and rodent hosts. In most instances, it is more convenient working with malarial parasites from nonhuman hosts because

**Table 7.2:** *In vitro* cultivation of stages of nonhuman Plasmodium spp.[a]

| Stage | Species | Basal medium[a] | Additional factors |
|---|---|---|---|
| Exoerythrocytic | P. berghei | L-15, MEM; NCTC-135 | Rodent liver cells, human embryonic lung or hepatoma cells |
| | P. cynomolgi | MEM | Primary hepatocytes |
| | P. fallax | Medium 199-LDGM | Turkey embryos |
| | P. yoellii | MEM | Human hepatoma cells |
| Erythrocytic | P. berghei | RPMI 1640 | |
| | P. chabaudi | BME; William's medium | Rhesus erythrocytes |
| | P. cynomolgi | | |
| | P. lophurae | Duck erythrocyte extract | |
| Sporogenic | P. berghei (oocysts) | RPMI 1640 | With or without insect cells, fetal bovine, and silkworm sera |
| | P. berghei (ookinetes) | MEM | |
| | P. gallinaceum | RPMI 1640 | Fetal bovine serum plus drosophila cells and Matrigel |
| | P. relictum (sporozoites and ookinetes) | Chicken serum and embryo extract | |

[a]Summary of the different media used for cultivation of the several species of the malaria parasite and their different stages.

they can be maintained *in vivo*, thereby allowing testing for infectivity of *in vitro*-cultured stages in the vertebrate host and providing an animal model for the study of the parasite in the human host.

## Exoerythrocytic Stages

Techniques for cultivation of the exoerythrocytic stages of avian malarial parasites *P. gallinaceum*, *P. lophurae*, and *P. fallax* a variety of tissue culture media supplemented with chicken serum (10–20%) and whole egg ultrafiltrate (5%) can be used to establish primary cultures of infected chicken embryo cells that could be kept for up to 7 months. *P. fallax* can be maintained in turkey embryos by successive transfer of infected tissue onto the chorioallanotic membrane of 2-week-old embryos. Once parasites were established in the embryos, infected brain tissue was removed, trypsinized to obtain a cell suspension, and transferred to flasks containing supplemented medium. These cultures could be maintained for two or three passages until heavy parasitism required addition of uninfected embryonic turkey brain cells or transfer of culture supernatant containing merozoites to uninfected normal turkey brain in culture. Primary cultures of hepatocytes from rhesus monkeys (*Macaca mulatta*) are used to support growth of several simian malarias (*P. cynomolgi, P. knowlesi, P. coatneyi,* and *P. inui*). Using sporozoites released from mosquito salivary glands, they found that less than 1% of the sporozoites survived to invade hepatocytes. Fungal contamination was a problem with cultured stages, requiring the addition of flucytosine to the culture medium. An arginine-deficient cell culture medium is used in some instances to prevent overgrowth of hepatocytes before parasite development can be observed *in vitro*. In a later study, Millet et al. used rhesus hepatocytes for cultivation of developmental stages of *P. fieldi* and *P. simiovale*, two parasites that infect macaques. They found that about 1 in $10^4$ sporozoites underwent development into schizonts in the hepatocytes. The rodent malarial parasite *P. berghei* from *in vivo*-infected livers can be maintained in primary cultures of rodent liver cells. These exoerythrocytic plasmodial stages retained their infectivity for rats. Human embryonic lung cells (W138) and human hepatoma cells (HepG2-A16) are used to cultivate the exoerythrocytic stage of *P. berghei*, with about 8% of the sporozoites developing within the hepatoma cells.

Two human hepatoma cell lines (huH-1 and huH-2) are used for exoerythrocytic development of *P. berghei* and *P. yoelii*. *P. berghei* would also develop in HeLa cells, but *P. yoelii* would not.

### Erythrocytic Stages

Erythrocytic development of a number of simian malarial parasites has been studied, including that of *P. knowlesi, P. cynomolgi, P. fragile, P. gonderi, P. coatneyi, P. inui, P. fieldi,* and *P. simiovale*. Some of these aforementioned malarias are nonhuman facsimiles of human malarias. Thus, *P. fragile* and *P. coatneyi* produce falciparum-like malaria in monkeys, *P. cynomolgi* produces vivax-like malaria, *P. inui* produces *P. malariae* type malaria, and *P. fieldi* and *P. simiovale* produce *P. ovale type* malaria. With few exceptions, these organisms have been maintained *in vitro* in their erythrocytic stages. Simian malarias. *P. fragile* was cultured using RPMI 1640 with a 1:1 mixture of rhesus and human AB sera and rhesus erythrocytes. A combination of rhesus and human sera was also effective in cultivation of *P. gonderi*. Human erythrocytes does not support development of simian malarial parasite, indicating host specificity. Cultivation was accomplished in candle jars, in plates or multiwell plates and sealed flasks, as well as in a continuous-flow system. Petri plate cultures in a candle jar would not support growth of *P. inui* in HEPES buffered RPMI 1640 with rhesus serum and erythrocytes.

A continuous-flow system was successful, however, with stages of *P. inui* formed after 35 days in culture infective for monkeys.

## Rodent Malaria

Among the rodent malarias, the erythrocytic stages of *P. berghei* and *P. chabaudi* have been cultivated *in vitro*. Static cultures of *P. berghei* are developed. In static cultures, conditions may rapidly develop that lead to inhibition of parasite growth and development. Stirring may facilitate rupture of erythrocytes as in passage of infected cells through host capillaries. The use of BME basal medium or BME plus William's medium E gave better growth of and incorporation of radioactive amino acids into *P. chabaudi* than did RPMI 1640 medium. No growth of simian or rodent malarias has been accomplished in cell-free systems.

## Avian Malaria

Among the avian malarias, the erythrocytic stage of *P. lophurae* has been cultivated *in vitro*. Parasitic stages of *P. lophurae* freed from host cells by immune lysis were grown extracellularly in duck erythrocyte extract. Degenerate forms of the parasite, reduced incorporation of labeled amino acids, and decreased number, size, and density of food vacuoles appeared with time (about 3 days) in cultured forms.

## Sporogonic Stages Ookinete Development

*In vitro* ookinete formation from *in vivo*-produced gametocytes of *P. berghei* in MEM and other tissue culture media was examined by Weiss and Vanderberg (96). Although MEM gave optimal results, the number of ookinetes formed was 1% or less of the number of macrogametocytes introduced. A better percentage of ookinete formation (up to 44%) can be obtained by comparing HEPES-buffered RPMI 1640 and MEM media, from *in vivo* and *in vitro*-produced *P. berghei* gametocytes. RPMI 1640 gives consistently higher ookinete yields than MEM. Development from gametocyte to oocyst occurred in an acellular medium consisting of RPMI 1640 or Grace's medium with 10 or 20% fetal bovine serum or 5% silkworm serum. The presence of insect cells (Aedes or Toxorhynchites spp.) increased by sixfold the number of oocysts produced compared to the acellular cultures. Cultures, however, did not develop beyond the oocyst stage.

### *Sporozoite Development*

*In vitro* development of sporozoites of *P. relictum*, an avian parasite, can be done in culture medium consisting of a phosphate and bicarbonate buffered basic salts solution, supplemented with glucose, amino acids, B vitamins, purines, and pyrimidines, plus chick serum and chicken embryo extract, in an atmosphere of 5% $CO_2$ and 95% air. High oxygen concentration was inhibitory for development of sporozoites. Development from gametocyte to mature oocyst with sporozoites but ceased after 5 days. In another series of experiments, stomachs of mosquitoes which had fed upon infected canaries and contained immature stages of oocysts was found to be dissected into a medium containing saline extract of pupae or adult mosquitoes at about 0.2%. Oocysts cultured for 48 or 96 hours produced sporozoites infective for canaries, demonstrating that a period of residence in the salivary gland of the mosquito is not essential for development of infectivity of sporozoites.

Grace's insect tissue culture medium supplemented with various kinds of sera (fetal bovine, chick, and rabbit), as well as insect hemolymph, chicken embryo extract, and different types of adult and embryonic insect tissue extracts and cells, can be used for *in vitro* development of sporozoites of *P. gallinaceum*, an avian parasite. Sporozoites were released from older (day 9), but not from younger oocysts. HEPES-buffered RPMI 1640 with 15% fetal bovine serum, supplemented with trehalose, hypoxanthine, and a lipoprotein-cholesterol mixture can be used to obtain sporozoites of *P. gallinaceum*. Matrigel, a basement membrane-like extract containing laminin and collagen type IV, served as a substrate with *D. melanogaster* L2 cells and a gas phase of 5% $CO_2$–5% $O_2$–90% $N_2$. Under these conditions, transformation of ookinetes into oocysts with subsequent development of sporozoites took place. Without Matrigel, the parasites clumped and only a small percentage of ookinetes developed. Table 7.2 presents a summary of the media used in cultivation of life cycle stages of the nonhuman malarial parasites that are dealt with in the present review.

## PROCEDURE FOR *IN VITRO* CULTIVATION AND MAINTENANCE OF *PLASMODIUM FALCIPARUM* CULTURE

### Preparation of Culture Medium for Cultivation of *Plasmodium falciparum*

**RPMI medium:** One packet of RPMI 1640 (containing 25 mM of HEPES buffer, glucose) dissolved in 960 mL of double distilled water. 40 µg/mL of gentamycin sulfate (1.2 mL of gentamycin/L) was to be added. This solution was passed through a Millipore filter of 0.22 µm porosity and store at 4°C as 96 mL aliquots in glass media bottle.

**Washing medium** (incomplete medium): 4.2 mL of 5% sodium bicarbonate (5 g of sodium bicarbonate was dissolved in 100 mL double distilled water and filtered through a Millipore filter of 0.22 μm porosity and store at 4°C) was added to 96 mL of stock RPMI 1640 media.

*Note:* The sodium bicarbonate should be added to the RPMI 1640 media only at the time of requirement and should be prepared afresh.

**Serum preparation:** O⁺ blood was collected in centrifuge tube without anticoagulant and kept at 4°C. Next day it was centrifuged at 10000 rpm for 20 minutes at 4°C. Serum was separated aseptically and kept in aliquots. The serum was inactivated by keeping it at 56°C water bath for half an hour.

*Note:* After inactivation the serum could be stored in deep freezer at –20°C/–70°C up to 6 months.

**Complete medium:** Normal inactivated O⁺ human serum (10 mL) was added to 90 mL of incomplete media.

*Preparation of erythrocytes (RBCs) for culture* O⁺ blood was collected in anticoagulant into centrifuge tubes. Then this was centrifuged at 1500 rpm for 10 minutes at room temperature. Plasma and buffy coat was removed with sterile Pasteur pipette. After this washing media was added, centrifuged at 1500 rpm for 10 minutes and supernatant was removed. This washing process was repeated thrice. Equal amount of complete media was added to the pellet and stored at 4°C.

*Note:* Prepared RBCs can be used up to 14 days for optimum parasite growth.

## Continuous Culture of Plasmodium falciparum

Initiation of culture suspension (50%) of infected cells with complete media (with 15% serum) was prepared. Appropriate amount of uninfected cells were added to get an initial parasitaemia of 0.5–1.0% and diluted with complete media to get 5% cell suspension (5% hematocrit). Culture was kept in $CO_2$ incubator at 37°C.

*Note:* Hematocrit is an important factor for the optimal growth of parasite.

**Monitoring culture growth:** After every 24-hour the media was removed using a sterile Pasteur pipette without disturbing the cells that settled down. Then the cells were mixed without frothing and a drop of blood was placed on the slide and a thin film was made. Fresh complete media (with 10% serum) was added, mixed properly, and kept back in the incubator. Thin film was stained and examined for parasitaemia. It was then compared with initial parasitaemia.

*Note:* Parasitaemia should not be kept above 2–3% in the culture, it should be subcultured.

**Smear preparation:** Culture (3.0 µL) was placed on a slide toward left side. The cells were smeared across the slide with the help of another slide, to get a thin film and dried the slide at room temperature. Slide was fixed by immersing in methanol for 30 seconds followed by drying. The slides were then stained with Field A stain for 15 seconds and washed with water to remove excess stain. The slide was then dried and consequently stained with Field B stain for 20 seconds and washed with water to remove the excess stain. It was then dried and observed under the microscope.

### Estimation of the Percentage of Erythrocytes Infected (% Parasitaemia) with *Plasmodium falciparum*

An area of stained thin blood film where the erythrocytes were evenly distributed, was observed using 100 × objective (under oil immersion). Approximately 100 erythrocytes in this area were counted. Without moving the slide, the number of infected erythrocytes amongst the 100 erythrocytes was also counted. The slide was moved randomly to adjacent fields and counting was continued as mentioned above. An equivalent of 1,000 erythocytes was counted. The counting was repeated twice for a total examination of three different parts of the slide, i.e. 3 areas 1000 cells. The mean number of infected RBCs per 1,000 RBCs was taken by dividing the infected RBCs by 3.

**Calculation**

A = Number of infected erythrocytes/1,000 erythrocytes

Percent infected erythrocytes (% parasitaemia) = A/10.

*Note:* If one erythrocyte contains ≥2 it is still counted as one infected erythrocyte.

**Subculturing (Passaging):** Old media was removed and freshly washed RBCs and complete media (with 10% serum) were added. For example, to 20 µL of infected RBCs with around 5% parasitaemia, 160 µL freshly washed RBCs (i.e. 80 µL RBCs) suspension (concentration of prasitaemia = 1%) and 2000 µL of complete media was added. Culture was dispensed to more vials.

*Note:* Culture should not be kept for more than a week in a glass vial, if growth was good, subculture or change the vial.

### Synchronization of *Plasmodium falciparum*

Malarial parasites in a continuous cycle of development consist of merozoites, ring-stages, trophozoites, and schizonts stages. Many species of Plasmodium undergo synchronous development in their natural hosts, but when *P. falciparum* is grown in *in vitro* culture, this synchrony is quite rapidly lost. Hence, a method for inducing synchrony in cultures of this parasite is a necessary first step. The most important thing for synchronization is to be sure that there should be enough ring-stage parasites. For tighter synchronization, it should be done several times until the ring-stage predominates in the cultures. Sorbitol destroys large parasites (trophozoites and schizonts) in erythrocytes.

**Procedure:** Sorbitol (5%) was prepared in distilled water and passed through a Millipore filter of 0.22 μm porosity. To 1 mL of the culture pellet, 9 mL of sorbitol was added and kept at 34 room temperature for 5 minutes. Supernatant was removed by centrifugation and pellet was washed thrice in complete media [washing procedure same as mentioned for preparation of erythrocytes (RBCs) for culture]. Freshly washed erythrocytes were added to the culture to setup new culture as described under continuous culture.

## Anticipated Results

After synchronization, ring-forms of *P. falciparum* persist as rings (Fig. 2.1.) in culture for about 18 hours. 24 hours later, the youngest rings became small trophozoites, and the oldest rings became schizonts (Fig. 2.2). Thus, at this stage the culture was still asynchronous to some extent. Approximately 6 hours later, the first generation of new merozoites invaded erythrocytes to become young rings. At this point a second sorbitol treatment allowed only these rings to survive and later these rings developed with a high degree of synchrony. Approximately 95% of the parasites were in the ring stage of development at 48 and 96 hours after sorbitol treatment-likewise, a high percentage of trophozoite and schizont stages was observed at 24, 72, and 120 hours. If the culture is not synchronized regularly, culture remains unsynchronized with mixed stages containing rings, trophozoites and schizonts (Fig. 2.3).

**Freezing and thawing of *Plasmodium falciparum*:** There are few methods for the cryopreservation of malaria parasite, viz. sorbitol method and glycerolyte method. Parasites frozen according to one method can be thawed using another method's thawing protocol.

*Note:* The culture selected for cryopresevation should contain more than 50% rings stages as higher stages get lysed in due course.

**Cryopreservation:** The cryopreservative was prepared by adding 28 mL glycerol to 72 mL of 4.2% sorbitol in normal saline. This solution was filtered through Millipore filter of 0.22 μm porosity. The infected blood was centrifuged at 1500 rpm for 10 minutes. The supernatant/plasma was removed. Equal volume of cryoprotectant was added to the cells, distributed in small screw cap vials (cryotubes) and frozen quickly by immersing in liquid nitrogen (–196°C). Vial was labelled with strain, date and % of rings.

**Revival of cryopreserved parasites:** The vial was taken out from the liquid nitrogen and thawed quickly in a 37°C water bath. Culture was then transferred to a centrifuge tube and centrifuged at 1500 rpm for 10 minutes at room temperature. The supernatant was removed and an equal volume of 3.5% NaCl was added (drop wise). This suspension was again centrifuged and the supernatant was removed. The pellet was washed twice with complete medium supplemented with 15% serum. After washing the cryopreserved cells, the culture was initiated by adding fresh washed erythrocytes as follows.

*Note:* After revival of cryopreserved parasites complete media should be used with 15% serum while in maintenance of continuous culture complete media with 10% serum can be used.

## Bibliography

1. Acharya, AS, Kaur, R, and Goel, AD (2017). Neglected tropical diseases-Challenges and opportunities in India. Indian Journal of Medical Specialities, 102–108.
2. Hotez, PJ, Molyneux, DH, Fenwick, A, Kumaresan, J, Sachs, SE, Sachs, JD, and Savioli, L (2007). Control of neglected tropical diseases. New England Journal of Medicine, 357(10), 1018–1027.

## EXPERIMENT 7.1

**Aim:** To study the *in vitro* antimalarial activity of the given sample by using 72 hours *in vitro* growth inhibition assay.

**Principle:** Malaria culture is the method to grow malaria parasites outside the body, i.e. in an *ex vivo* environment. The *in vitro* growth inhibition assay measures the capacity of the antimalarial agent under study to limit red blood cell (RBC) invasion and/or intra-RBC growth of *P. falciparum* in a malarial culture maintained *ex vivo*. Several versions of this assay have been used in the preclinical phases of malaria vaccine development.

### Requirements

*Strain*: *Plasmodium falciparum* line 3D7 (MRA-102), line W2 (MRA-157), as well as artemisinin-resistant *P. falciparum* strains (MRA-1236 and MRA-1240).

*Chemicals*: Purified erythrocytes [or human blood type O$^+$ in CPD (citrate-phosphate-dextrose) adenine], malaria culture medium (MCM), Tris, albumax II, RPMI 1640, gentamicin, 1 M HEPES [4-(2-hydroxyethyl)-1-piperazineethanesulfonic acid], Hanks' balanced salt solution, acridine orange (10 µg/mL) or Giemsa 5%, [3H] hypoxanthine and sodium-bi-carbonate.

*Equipment*: Incubator (37°C), glass desiccator (e.g. candle jar), cell culture flask, candles, centrifuge, sterile pipettes, sterile tubes, glass slides and coverslips, microscope, fluorescence or light, cell harvester and liquid scintillating counter.

### Procedure

1. Prepare malaria culture medium and Tris-buffered Hanks' (TH) for washing cells. For growing parasites from patient blood, use 10 g of albumax for 1 liter of complete MCM. The vast majority of cultures will survive at least 2 weeks. It is also important to avoid serum in the culture for preparation of crude parasite antigen.

2. *In vitro* cultures in tissue-culture flasks

    i. Wash the erythrocytes 3 times in TH or RPMI 1640 to remove CPD, serum, and leukocytes if present. Dilute to 5% hematocrit with cMCM in small flasks of 25 cm$^2$ (0.2 mL of packed cells to 4 mL of cMCM) or in 75 cm$^2$ flasks (1.0–20 mL).

    ii. Add parasites to maintain an appropriate parasitaemia.

   iii. Put the flask in a candle jar and loosen the cover. Produce low oxygen by burnt out candle and place the jar at 37°C.

   iv. Replace the MCM every day (not necessary the day after subcultivation). Subculture the cultures 2 times/week.

3. *Subcultivation*:

   i. Stain a drop of the culture with acridine orange (10 µg/mL) on a glass slide and put on a coverslip or by Giemsa staining of a thin smear.

   ii. Count the parasitaemia (i.e. the percentage of infected cells).

   iii. Prepare freshly washed O$^+$ blood in cMCM (5% hematocrit) and add it to the culture to obtain a parasitaemia of not more than 1%, preferably 0.1–0.5% if two cycles until next subculturing, 0.5–1% if one cycle. Parasitaemia should never exceed 15%.

4. *Antimalarial assay*:

   i. The test compounds are initially dissolved in DMSO and diluted 400-fold in RPMI 1640 culture medium supplemented with 25 mM Tris-buffered Hanks', 32 mM $NaHCO_3$, and 10% human plasma. These solutions are subsequently serially diluted to a twofold different concentrations.

   ii. The parasites were preexposed to the compounds for 48 hours and incubated at 37°C with 5% $O_2$, 5% $CO_2$, and 90% $N_2$ prior to the addition of r3H1-hypoxanthine. After a further incubation for 18 hours, parasite DNA was harvested from each microtiter well using a cell harvester onto glass filters.

   iii. Uptake of [3H] hypoxanthine was measured with a liquid scintillation counter. Concentration-response data were analyzed by a logistic dose-response model, and the IC50 values (50% inhibitory concentration) for each compound were calculated.

**Calculation:** IC50 is the drug concentration causing 50% inhibition of the desired activity.

## Bibliography

1. Lalitha, MK (2004). Manual on antimicrobial susceptibility testing. Performance standards for antimicrobial testing: Twelfth Informational Supplement, 56238, 454–456.

2. Wachino, JI, Kimura, K, Yamada, K, Jin, W, and Arakawa, Y (2014). Evaluation of Disk Potentiation Test Using Kirby-Bauer Disks Containing High-Dosage Fosfomycin and Glucose-6-Phosphate To Detect Production of Glutathione S-Transferase Responsible for Fosfomycin Resistance. Journal of Clinical Microbiology, 52(10), 3827–3828.

### EXPERIMENT 7.2

**Aim:** To study the *in vitro* antimalarial activity of the given sample by using hemozoin-based colorimetric method.

**Principle:** During the development and proliferation stage in host erythrocytes, the malaria parasites degrade hemoglobin for use as a major source of amino acids. This is accompanied by the release of free heme. Heme is a prosthetic group that consists of an iron atom contained in the center of a heterocyclic porphyrin ring. Free heme is oxidatively active and toxic for the malarial parasites, and can even cause parasite death, so the parasites convert it into an insoluble crystalline form called hemozoin. Thus, presence of hemozoin in blood in indicative of presence of malaria and consequently hemozoin is often called malaria pigment. Therefore, a simple and inexpensive *in vitro* assay was developed based on the colorimetric quantification of hemozoin in infected red blood cells to evaluate the anti-malarial activity of drugs.

## Requirements

*Chemicals*: Standard antimalarial stock solution, test sample solution, hemin chloride (heme), RPMI 1640 medium, hypoxanthine, gentamycin and albumax II.

*Strain*: *Plasmodium falciparum* K1 and 9A strains.

*Equipment*: Autoclave, incubator and water bath and 96-well microplate.

*Glasswares*: Conical flasks, beakers, pipettes, petri dishes measuring cylinder and glass rod.

## Procedure

1. Plasmodium cultivation: *Plasmodium falciparum* K1 and 9A strains are maintained *in vitro* continuous culture.

   i. The culture medium consisted of RPMI 1640 supplemented with 0.025 mg/mL gentamicin, 0.01 mM hypoxanthine, 23.8 mM $NaHCO_3$, 11 mM glucose and 0.5% albumax II, and adjusted to a pH of 7.3–7.4.

   ii. The parasites are cultured and maintained in a tissue culture flask with complete culture medium containing 5% human erythrocytes. The parasite density is maintained at about 1.5% parasitaemia under 20% $CO_2$ and $O_2$ (<0.1%) 37°C. Every 2 days, transfer the infected erythrocytes into fresh medium containing 5% human erythrocyte.

iii. The level of parasitaemia is determined by light microscopy on a Giemsa-stained thin blood smear, and parasitized erythrocytes were diluted when parasitaemia was higher than 5% in erythrocytes contained at 5% in culture medium, in order to lower parasitaemia and allow continuous growth.

iv. Parasite culture is diluted with fresh uninfected erythrocytes and culture medium to achieve a starting parasitaemia of 2% and a hematocrit of 5%. This final parasite culture is immediately used for antimalarial assay.

2. Stocks of drugs are prepared in dimethyl sulphoxide or phosphate buffer saline (for chloroquine) and were then serially diluted with complete culture medium. To each well of a microplate, 10 µL of serially diluted drug solution is added into 200 µL of final asynchronous parasite culture. Dimethyl sulphoxide or phosphate buffer saline are also tested by adding a similar amount to control wells.

3. The microplates are cultured for 72 hours under the conditions as described below.

A culture of the *P. falciparum* K1 strain was serially diluted with uninfected erythrocytes in complete medium to yield a hematocrit of 5% and parasitaemia ranging from 0 to 10%. The serial culture containing 200 µL is prepared independently in triplicate in microtubes, followed by the addition of 800 µL of 2.5% sodium dodecyl sulphate in 0.1 M sodium bicarbonate pH 8.8, then the samples are mixed at room temperature for 15 minutes. After centrifugation at 13,000 rpm for 10 minutes, the supernatant is removed. The pellet is washed twice with 800 µL of 2.5% sodium dodecyl sulfate in 0.1 M sodium bicarbonate (pH 8.8), then 200 µL of 5% sodium dodecyl sulfate is added to 50 mM NaOH to convert the hemozoin into heme. After incubation at room temperature for 30 minutes, the sample (200 µL) was transferred to a 96-well microplate and scanned at 405/750 nm (A405 nm minus A750 nm) using an IMark microplate reader. After the background absorbance of hemozoin is purified of uninfected erythrocytes (5% hematocrit) then subtracted, the amount of hemozoin in the infected erythrocytes was presented as the absorbance at 405/750 nm and then plotted against parasitaemia.

4. The hemozoin of infected erythrocytes is extracted, purified, and quantified, as described above. The 50% inhibitory concentration (IC50) value is calculated.

## Observation

| S. no. | Absorbance of control | Absorbance of test | Absorbance of standard |
|--------|-----------------------|--------------------|------------------------|
| 1.     |                       |                    |                        |
| 2.     |                       |                    |                        |
| 3.     |                       |                    |                        |

**Calculation:** The percentage inhibition of hemozoin formation was calculated as follows:

$$\text{Percentage antimalarial activity} = \frac{(\text{Abs control} - \text{Abs sample})}{\text{Abs control}} \times 100$$

where,  Abs control—absorbance of control

Abs sample—absorbance of sample

## Bibliography

1. Brown, DF, Wootton, M, and Howe, RA (2016). Antimicrobial susceptibility testing breakpoints and methods from BSAC to EUCAST. Journal of Antimicrobial Chemotherapy, 71(1), 3–5.
2. Lalitha, MK (2004). Manual on antimicrobial susceptibility testing. Performance standards for antimicrobial testing: Twelfth Informational Supplement, 56238, 454–456.
3. Piddock, LJ (1990). Techniques used for the determination of antimicrobial resistance and sensitivity in bacteria. Journal of Applied Bacteriology, 68(4), 307–318.

## EXPERIMENT 7.3

**Aim:** To study the *in vitro* antimalarial activity of the given sample by using candle jar method.

**Principle:** Infected human red blood cells are incubated in a culture dish or flask at 37°C together with a nutrient medium and plasma, serum or serum substitutes. A special feature of the incubation is the special gas mixture of mostly nitrogen (93% nitrogen, 4% carbon dioxide and 3% oxygen) allowing the parasites to grow at 37°C in a cell incubator. An alternative to gasing the cultures with the exact gas mixture, is the use of a candle jar. The candle jar is an airtight container in which the cultures and a lit candle are placed. The burning candle consumes some of the oxygen and produces carbon dioxide ($CO_2$), which acts as a fire extinguisher. Carbon dioxide content in fresh air varies between 0.036% and 0.039%, at approximately 5% $CO_2$ concentration the candle stops burning. The number of parasites increased by a factor 5 approximately every 48 hours (= one cycle). The parasitaemia can be determined via blood film, to keep it within the wanted limits the culture can be thinned out with healthy red blood cells.

### Requirements

*Chemicals:* Standard antimicrobial stock solution, test sample solution, RPMI-1640 medium, type A⁺ healthy blood sample, standard drug and Panotico Rapido Kit/JSB (Jaswant Singh–Bhattacharji) stain/Giemsa stain for staining.

*Strain:* Chloroquine-resistant (CQR) *Plasmodium falciparum* W2 clone and K1 strain.

*Equipment:* Candle jar and 96-well plate.

*Glasswares:* Conical flasks, beakers, measuring cylinder and glass rod, sterile graduated pipettes of 10 mL, 5 mL, 2 mL and 1 mL, sterile capped 7.5 × 1.3 cm tubes/small screw-capped bottles, and Pasteur pipettes.

### Procedure

1. Take CQR *Plasmodium falciparum* W2 clone and K1 strain in a candle jar. Cultivate the parasites in type A⁺ erythrocytes using culture medium (Roswell Park Memorial Institute or RPMI-1640) enriched with 10% human serum (complete medium) and maintained at 37°C under an atmosphere of 5% carbon dioxide, 5% oxygen and 90% nitrogen.

2. Monitor parasite growth every 24 hours during the daily refreshing of culture medium and calculate parasitaemia as a percentage based on the viable parasitic forms observed by counting at least 2000 erythrocytes.

3. Parasite quantification by optical microscopy is a traditional and reliable technique in the performance of *in vitro* antiplasmodial assays.

4. Dissolve the test substance in suitable solvent to provide a stock solution (5.0 mg/mL). Prepare dilutions of the test solutions by diluting stock solution in RPMI-1640 culture medium.

5. Introduce 20 µL of each dilution test solution into the wells of a 96-well plate. Add suspension of sorbitol-synchronized, parasitized red blood cells (pRBCs) adjusted to 1% parasitaemia and 3% hematocrit in complete medium (180 µL/well).

6. Screen sample at final (well) concentrations of 50 and 5.0 µg/mL. Prepare negative control with a suspension of pRBCs and 1% DMSO. Chloroquine is used as positive control.

7. Incubate the test plates at 37°C for 48 hours in a candle jar. After 48 hours, prepare thin blood smears of the contents of each well were stained with Panotico Rapido Kit/JSB (Jaswant Singh–Bhattacharji) stain/Giemsa stain for evaluation of the parasitaemia using an optical microscope.

**Calculation:** The parasitaemia was expressed as a percentage of the viable erythrocytic parasite forms observed in 2000 RBCs. Parasite inhibition was expressed as a percentage of the growth of untreated (negative) controls. All assays were performed in triplicate.

## Bibliography

1. Lima RBS, Rocha e Silva LF, Melo MRS, et al. (2015). *In vitro* and *in vivo* antimalarial activity of plants from the Brazilian Amazon. Malaria Journal,14, 508.

2. Ye, Z, and Dyke, KV (2015). Antimalarial Activity of Various Bisbenzylisoquinoline and Aporphine-Benzylisoquinoline Alkaloids and their Structure-Activity Relationships against Chloroquine-Sensitive and Resistant Plasmodium falciparum Malaria *in vitro*. Malaria Contr Elimination, 4, 137.

## EXPERIMENT 7.4

**Aim:** To study the *in vitro* activity of the given sample against leishmaniasis using leishmanicidal assay.

**Principle:** The leishmania life cycle consists of two developmental forms—promastigotes, flagellated extracellular parasites of the digestive tract of sand flies, and amastigotes, nonflagellated, nonmotile stages that is more sensitive and live inside parasitophorous vacuoles in macrophages of mammalian hosts. The present study describes the evaluation of anti-leishmania activity of test compounds on both Leishmania stages.

### Requirements

*Chemicals:* Standard antimicrobial stock solution, test sample solution, agar media, overnight broth culture of test and control organisms, sterile phosphate buffer saline (PBS) and tissue culture medium M-199, 4-(2-hydroxyethyl)-1-piperazineethanesulfonic acid (HEPEs), heat inactivated fetal bovine serum (HIFBS) methanol, DMSO and standard drug.

*Equipment:* Autoclave, incubator and water bath 96-well microplate.

*Glasswares:* Conical flasks, beakers, measuring cylinder and glass rod sterile graduated pipettes of 10 mL, 5 mL, 2 mL and 1 mL, sterile capped 7.5 × 1.3 cm tubes/small screw-capped bottles, Pasteur pipettes, a suitable rack to hold 22 tubes in two rows, i.e. 11 tubes in each row.

### Procedure

1. Leishmanial promastigotes are cultured in sterile 25 cm$^2$ tissue culture flask in tissue culture medium M-199 supplemented with 25 mM HEPES and 10% HIFBS at 25°C.

2. Parasites are centriguged at 3000 rpm, diluted in minimum volume of PBS and are counted with the help of improved Neubauer chamber under a microscope.

3. Parasites are then diluted with the fresh medium to a final concentration of 2.0 × 10$^6$ parasites mL$^{-1}$.

4. 1.0 mg of compound is dissolved in 50 μL of absolute methanol or DMSO and the volume is made up to 1.0 mL with the culture medium.

5. In a 96-well microtiter plate, 90 μL of the parasite culture (2.0 × 10$^6$ parasites mL$^{-1}$) is placed and 10 μL containing various concentrations of the experimental compound is added in the culture. Add 10 μL of phosphate buffered saline, pH 7.2 to the reaction mixture.

6. Methanol/0.5% DMSO is added as negative control while amphotericin B, and pentamidine (to a final concentration of 1.0 mg mL$^{-1}$) are added separately as positive control.

7. The plates are incubated at 25°C in the dark for 3–5 days during which control organisms multiply 3–6 times. The culture is examined microscopically on an improved Neubauer chamber and ED50 value of compounds possessing antileishmanial activity is calculated.

**Calculation:** Effective dose 50 (ED50) or median effective dose is the pharmacological term defining the dose or amount of drug that produces a therapeutic response or desired effect in 50% of the subjects taking it.

## Bibliography

1. Lalitha, MK (2004). Manual on antimicrobial susceptibility testing. Performance standards for antimicrobial testing: Twelfth Informational Supplement, 56238, 454–456.

2. Wiegand, I, Hilpert, K and Hancock, RE (2008). Agar and broth dilution methods to determine the minimal inhibitory concentration (MIC) of antimicrobial substances. Nature Protocols, 3(2), 163–175.

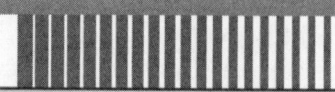

# CHAPTER 8

# *In vitro* Anticancer Assay

**Cancer** is an umbrella term covering a plethora of conditions characterized by unscheduled and uncontrolled cellular proliferation and abnormal cell growth with the potential to invade or spread to other parts of the body.

### Hallmarks of Cancer Cell

- *Uncontrolled growth and proliferation*: Cancer cells do not respond to many of the signals that control cellular growth and death. Cancer cells even evade programmed cell death, despite the fact that their multiple abnormalities would normally make them prime targets for apoptosis.
- *Invasiveness*: Malignant cells generally secrete proteases that digest extracellular matrix components, allowing the cancer cells to invade adjacent normal tissues.
- *Metastasis*: In the late stages of cancer, cells break through normal tissue boundaries and metastasize (spread) to new sites in the body.
- *Angiogenesis*: Cancer cells secrete growth factors that promote the formation of new blood vessels (angiogenesis). Angiogenesis is needed to support the growth of a tumor beyond the size of about a million cells, at which point new blood vessels are required to supply oxygen and nutrients to the proliferating tumor cells.

### Etiology of Cancer

Tobacco smoking is linked with tobacco use and cancer in the lung, larynx, head, neck, stomach, bladder, kidney, esophagus and pancreas. Tobacco smoke contains over fifty known carcinogens, including nitrosamines and polycyclic aromatic hydrocarbons. Diet, physical inactivity, and obesity are related to approximately 30–35% of cancer deaths. For example, a high-salt diet is linked to gastric cancer, aflatoxin B1, a frequent food contaminate with liver cancer, and betel nut chewing with oral cancer.

Oncovirus viruses are the usual infectious agents that can cause cancer. These include human papillomavirus implicated in cervical carcinoma, Epstein-Barr virus in B-cell lymphoproliferative disease and nasopharyngeal carcinoma, human herpes virus-8 in Kaposi's sarcoma and primary effusion lymphomas, hepatitis B, and hepatitis C viruses in hepatocellular carcinoma and Human T-cell leukemia virus-1 in T-cell leukemias. Bacterial infection may also increase the risk of cancer, as seen in *Helicobacter pylori*-induced gastric carcinoma. Parasitic infections strongly associated with cancer include *Schistosoma haematobium* induced squamous cell carcinoma of the bladder and liver flukes, *Opisthorchis viverrini* and *Clonorchis sinensis* induced cholangiocarcinoma.

Up to 10% of invasive cancers are related to radiation exposure, including both ionizing radiation and nonionizing ultraviolet radiation. Some substances cause cancer primarily through their physical, rather than chemical, effects on cells. A prominent example of this is prolonged exposure to asbestos, synthetic asbestos-like fibers such as wollastonite, attapulgite, glass wool, and rock wool. Nonfibrous particulate materials that cause cancer include powdered metallic cobalt and nickel, and crystalline silica (quartz, cristobalite, and tridymite).

## Pathophysiology of Cancer

Healthy cells have a specific size, structure, function and growth rate that best serves the needs of the tissues they compose. Cancer cells differ from normal cells in size, structure, function, and growth rate. These malignant cells lack the normal controls of growth seen in healthy cells, and grow uncontrollably. This uncontrolled growth allows the cancer cells to invade adjacent structures and then destroy surrounding tissues and organs. Malignant cells may also metastasize to other areas of the body through the cardiovascular or lymphatic systems. This uncontrolled growth and spread of cancer cells can eventually interfere with one or more of a person's vital organs or functions and possibly lead to death. The primary sites of cancer metastasis are bone, lymph nodes, liver, lungs, and brain human cancer-derived cell lines are the most widely used models to study the biology of cancer and to test hypotheses to improve cancer treatment.

## Cancer Cell Lines

Cancer cell lines are defined as cancer cells that keep dividing and growing over time, under certain conditions in a laboratory. They are used in research

**Table 8.1:** Examples of some cancer cell lines

| S. no. | Cancer cell lines | Associated cancer |
|--------|-------------------|-------------------|
| 1. | SH-SY5Y | Human neuroblastoma |
| 2. | Hep G2 | Human Caucasian hepatocyte carcinoma |
| 3. | 293 (also known as HEK 293) | Human embryo kidney |
| 4. | RAW 264.7 | Mouse monocyte macrophage |
| 5. | HeLa | Human cervix epitheloid carcinoma |
| 6. | MRC-5 (PD 19) | Human foetal lung |
| 7. | A2780 | Human ovarian carcinoma |
| 8. | CACO-2 | Human Caucasian colon adenocarcinoma |
| 9. | THP 1 | Human monocytic leukemia |
| 10. | A549 | Human Caucasian lung carcinoma |

to study the biology of cancer and to test cancer treatments. Human cancer-derived cell lines are fundamental models used in laboratories to study the biology of cancer, and to test the therapeutic efficacy of anticancer agents. HeLa was the first cultured cancer line. It was derived from cervical cancer cells taken from Henrietta Lacks in 1951. Since then, hundreds of cancer cell lines have been established and propagated either *in vitro* as monolayer cultures or *in vivo* as xenografts in mice. Table 8.1 enlists examples of some popular cancer cell lines used in preclinical studies.

## Bibliography

1. Hundie, GB, Woldemeskel, D, and Gessesse, A (2017). Correction: Evaluation of Direct Colorimetric MTT Assay for Rapid Detection of Rifampicin and Isoniazid Resistance in *Mycobacterium Tuberculosis*. PloS One, 12(2), e0171964.

2. Karp, G (2010). Cell and Molecular Biology: Concepts and Experiments 6th Edition with Plus Set. John Wiley & Son. 650–682.

3. Yilmaz, M, and Christofori, G (2009). EMT, the cytoskeleton, and cancer cell invasion. Cancer and Metastasis Reviews, 28(1–2), 15–33.

## EXPERIMENT 8.1

**Aim:** To study the *in vitro* antimitotic potential of the given sample using *Allium cepa* root tip assay.

**Principle:** Higher plants such as *Allium cepa* are accepted as admirable genetic models to evaluate genotoxic effects such as chromosome aberrations and disturbances in the mitotic cycle. *Allium cepa* assay enables the assessment of mitotic index and chromosome aberration. Mitotic index is characterized by the total number of dividing cells in cell cycle. It is used as an indicator of cell proliferation biomarkers which measures the proportion of cells in the mitotic phase of the cell cycle. Hence, the decrease in the mitotic index of *Allium cepa* meristematic cells could be interpreted as cellular death. Mitotic index (MI) is an indirect measure of cell proliferation that has been demonstrated to be a strong predictor of outcome for several anticancer treatments.

### Requirements

*Chemicals*: Standard drug solution (vincristine), test sample solution, 1 N hydrochloric acid solution, acetic acid, alcohol, aceto-orcein or toluidine blue.

*Equipment*: Microscope.

*Glasswares*: Beakers, pipettes, measuring cylinder, glass rod, slides and coverslips.

### Procedure

1. Grow the *A. cepa* bulbs in tap water at room temperature. The *A. cepa* bulbs will sprout in water after approximately 48 hours if constantly maintained at room temperature. The bulbs that developed uniform root are selected for the study. Divide the bulbs into test, positive control (standard treated group) and control groups (3 bulbs per group).
2. Dip the roots of the test and positive control groups in varying concentrations of test and standard drugs for 48 hours. Use water for dilution as well as a control and vincristine as a standard for study.
3. Change the solutions daily, harvest root tips from each bulb, fixed in Carnoy's fixative (1:3 acetic acid: alcohol) for 24 hours.
4. After pretreatment, wash the root tips a few times with distilled water. Then hydrolyze with 1 N HCl at 60–70°C for 5 minutes. After hydrolysis, again wash the roots.
5. Then cut and place, about 1–2 mm of the root tips on the slide. Drop a small drop of aceto-orcein (toluidine blue can be used as an alternative) on the root tip and leave the slide undisturbed for 2 minutes. Squash the

root tip and add another small drop of aceto-orcein and leave the slide undisturbed for another 2 minutes.

6. Carefully lower the coverslip on to avoid air bubbles and seal the sides of the slides with clear fingernail polish.

7. Observe the slides under the light microscope at 400× and 630× magnification. Photomicrographs the slides. A minimum of 100 cells per slide are used for the purpose of analysis (observe a minimum of nine slides for each treatment).

8. Replicate the experiment 3 times with three roots for each replicate therefore, nine slides are prepared for each treatment group.

9. Calculate the mitotic index for all the three groups.

**Calculation:** Mitotic index is calculated as follows:

$$\text{Mitotic index} = \frac{\text{Number of dividing or mitotic cells}}{\text{Total number of cells}} \times 100$$

## Observation

Example of photomicrograph:

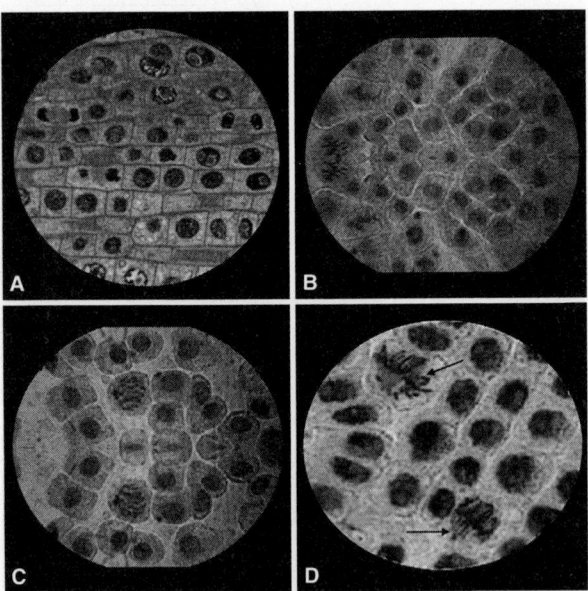

**Fig. 8.1A to D:** *Allium cepa* root meristem cells in mitotic dividing stage (Patel et al., 2013). (A) Normal cells in telophase mitotic dividing stage; (B and C) abnormal dividing cells in standard drug treated group showing multipolarity and sticky chromosome; (D) normal as well as few abnormal dividing cells in test treated root showing sticky and vagrant chromosome.

## Bibliography

1. Nefic, H, Musanovic, J, Metovic, A, and Kurteshi, K (2013). Chromosomal and Nuclear Alterations in Root Tip Cells of Allium Cepa L. Induced by Alprazolam. Medical Archives, 67(6), 388–392.

2. Patel, A, Bigoniya, P, Singh, CS, and Patel, NS (2013). Radioprotective and cytoprotective activity of *Tinospora cordifolia* stem enriched extract containing cordifolioside-A. Indian Journal of Pharmacology, 45(3), 237.

3. Yuet Ping, K, Darah, I, Yusuf, UK, Yeng, C, and Sasidharan, S (2012). Genotoxicity of *Euphorbia hirta*: an Allium cepa assay. Molecules, 17(7), 7782–7791.

**Aim:** To study the *in vitro* antimitotic potential of the given sample using germination assay.

**Principle:** Mitotic index is characterized by the total number of dividing cells in cell cycle. It is used as an indicator of cell proliferation biomarkers which measures the proportion of cells in the mitotic phase of the cell cycle. Hence, the decrease in the mitotic index of root tip meristematic cells could be interpreted as cellular death. Mitotic index (MI) is an indirect measure of cell proliferation that has been demonstrated to be a strong predictor of outcome for several anticancers treatments.

## Requirements

*Chemicals*: Standard drug solution (vincristine), test sample solution, 1 N hydrochloric acid solution, acetic acid, alcohol, aceto-orcein or toluidine blue.

*Equipment*: Microscope, 24-well plate.

*Glasswares*: Beakers, pipettes, measuring cylinder, glass rod, slides and coverslips.

## Procedure

1. Take 200–500 µL of aqueous solution of graded doses of the sample in 24-well plate and add equal weight dry seeds of *Cicer arietinum* one to each microtitre well and close the plate with lid and leave at room temperature for 24 hours for imbibition of water.

2. At the end of the test period (24 hours), dry and weigh the seeds. For morphological studies, extend the time of sprouting to either 72 hours or 96 hours, and take photographs.

3. Change the solutions daily and after 48 hours, harvest root tips from each bulb, fixed in Carnoy's fixative (1:3 acetic acid: alcohol) for 24 hours.

4. After pretreatment, wash the root tips a few times with distilled water. Then hydrolyze with 1 N HCl at 60–70°C for 5 minutes. After hydrolysis, again wash the roots.

5. Then cut and place, about 1–2 mm of the root tips on the slide. Drop a small drop of aceto-orcein (toluidine blue can be used as an alternative) on the root tip and leave the slide undisturbed for 2 minutes. Squash the root tip and add another small drop of aceto-orcein and leave the slide undisturbed for another 2 minutes.

6. Carefully lower the coverslip on to avoid air bubbles and seal the sides of the slides with clear fingernail polish.
7. Observe the slides under the light microscope at 400× and 630× magnification. Photomicrograph the slides. A minimum of 100 cells per slide are used for the purpose of analysis (observe a minimum of nine slides for each treatment).
8. Replicate the experiment 3 times with three roots for each replicate therefore, nine slides are prepared for each treatment group.
9. Calculate the mitotic index for all the three groups.

## Observation

Example of sprouting assay (Fig. 8.2):

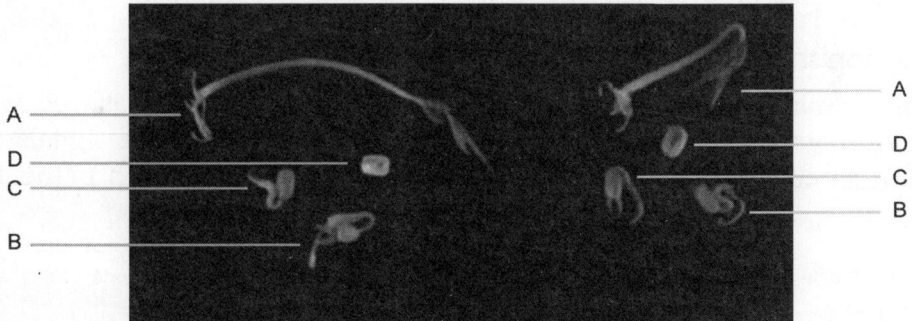

**Fig. 8.2:** Germination of green-gram seeds in water in the presence and absence of test sample is shown in the figure. The sprouted seed had developed roots, shoot and two leaves (A). In contrast, seeds that sprouted in the presence of 10 µL test sample had reduced growth with shortened shoot and small leaves (B), with no visible roots. At 20 µL concentration inhibition of growth was much more pronounced, and at 100 µL, inhibition of germination was complete with no visible sprouting (C and D). These morphological observations indicate the dose dependence of inhibition. (Murthy et al., 2011).

**Calculation:** Mitotic index is calculated as follows:

$$\text{Mitotic index} = \frac{\text{Number of dividing or mitotic cells}}{\text{Total number of cells}} \times 100$$

## Bibliography

1. Murthy, GS, Francis, TP, Singh, CR, Nagendra, HG, and Naik, C (2011). An assay for screening anti-mitotic activity of herbal extracts. Current Science (00113891), 100(9).

2. Nefic, H, Musanovic, J, Metovic, A, and Kurteshi, K (2013). Chromosomal and Nuclear Alterations in Root Tip Cells of Allium Cepa L. Induced by Alprazolam. Medical Archives, 67(6), 388–392.

3. Yuet Ping, K, Darah, I, Yusuf, UK, Yeng, C, and Sasidharan, S (2012). Genotoxicity of *Euphorbia hirta*: an Allium cepa assay. Molecules, 17(7), 7782–7791.

## *IN VITRO* APOPTOSIS ASSAY

Cell death has an important role in many human diseases, and strategies aimed at modulating the associated pathways have been successfully applied to treat various disorders. Indeed, several clinically promising cytotoxic and cytoprotective agents with potential applications in cancer, ischemic and neurodegenerative diseases have recently been identified based on appropriate cell death assays.

## Mechanism of Apoptosis

The two main pathways of apoptosis are extrinsic and intrinsic as well as a perforin/granzyme pathway. Each requires specific triggering signals to begin an energy-dependent cascade of molecular events. Each pathway

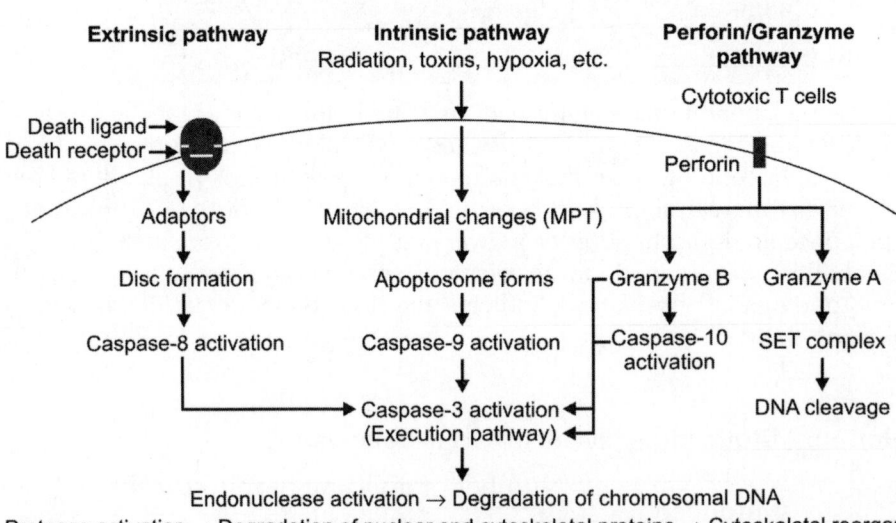

**Fig. 8.3:** Pathways of apoptosis

activates its own initiator caspase (8, 9, 10) which in turn will activate the executioner caspase-3. However, granzyme A works in a caspase-independent fashion. The execution pathway results in characteristic cytomorphological features including cell shrinkage, chromatin condensation, formation of cytoplasmic blebs and apoptotic bodies and finally phagocytosis of the apoptotic bodies by adjacent parenchymal cells, neoplastic cells, or macrophages. Figure 8.3 describes schematic representation of apoptotic events that occurs in the three separate pathways.

## Bibliography

1. Elmore, S (2007). Apoptosis: a review of programmed cell death. Toxicologic Pathology, 35(4), 495–516.
2. Marino, G, Niso-Santano, M, Baehrecke, EH, and Kroemer, G (2014). Self-consumption: the interplay of autophagy and apoptosis. Nature reviews. Molecular Cell Biology, 15(2), 81.
3. Mukhopadhyay, S, Panda, PK, Sinha, N, Das, DN, and Bhutia, SK (2014). Autophagy and apoptosis: where do they meet?. Apoptosis, 19(4), 555–566.

**Aim:** To study the *in vitro* MTS cytotoxicity assays.

**Principle:** The assay can be used for the measurement of cell proliferation in response to growth factors, cytokines, mitogens, nutrients, etc. It can also be used for the analysis of cytotoxic compounds like anticancer drugs and many other toxic agents and pharmaceutical compounds. MTS cell proliferation assay is a colorimetric method for sensitive quantification of viable cells in proliferation and cytotoxicity assay. The assay is based on the reduction of MTS tetrazolium compound by viable cells to generate a colored formazan product that is soluble in cell culture media. This conversion is thought to be carried out by NAD(P)H-dependent dehydrogenase enzymes in metabolically active cells. The formazan dye produced by viable cells can be quantified by measuring the absorbance at 490–500 nm.

## Requirements

*Chemicals*: Standard drug solution (vincristine), test sample solution, MTS [3-(4,5-dimethylthiazol-2-yl)-5-(3-carboxymethoxyphenyl)-2-(4-sulfophenyl)-2H-tetrazolium, inner salt], Dulbecco's phosphate-buffered saline (DPBS), and phenazine ethosulfate (PES).

*Equipment*: 96-well plate.

*Glasswares*: Beakers, pipettes, measuring cylinder, glass rod, slides, and coverslips.

## Procedure

**Reagent preparation:** MTS solution (containing PES)

1. Dissolve MTS powder in DPBS to 2 mg/mL to produce a clear golden-yellow solution.
2. Dissolve PES powder in MTS solution to 0.21 mg/mL.
3. Adjust to pH 6.0–6.5 using 1 N HCl.
4. Filter-sterilize through a 0.2 μm filter into a sterile, light protected container.
5. Store the MTS solution containing PES protected from light at 4°C for frequent use or at –20°C for long term storage.

## MTS Assay Protocol

1. Prepare cells and test compounds in 96-well plates containing a final volume of 100 μL/well. An optional set of wells can be prepared with medium only for background subtraction.

2. Incubate for desired period of exposure.
3. Add 20 μL MTS solution containing PES to each well (final concentration of MTS will be 0.33 mg/mL).
4. Incubate 1–4 hours at 37°C.
5. Record absorbance at 490 nm.

One of the advantages of the tetrazolium assays that produce an aqueous soluble formazan is that absorbance can be recorded form the assay plates periodically during early stages of incubation. Multiple readings may assist during assay development; but caution should be taken to return the plates to the incubator between readings to maintain a nearly constant environment. Extended incubations with the tetrazolium reagent beyond 4 hours should be avoided.

## Observation

| S. no. | Absorbance of control | Absorbance of test | Absorbance of standard |
|--------|----------------------|--------------------|------------------------|
| 1. | | | |
| 2. | | | |
| 3. | | | |

**Calculation:** The percentage cytotoxic potential is calculated as follows:

$$\text{Percentage cytotoxic potential} = \frac{(\text{Abs control} - \text{Abs sample})}{\text{Abs control}} \times 100$$

where,  Abs control—absorbance of control (the control represents 100% viability)

Abs sample—absorbance of sample

## Bibliography

1. Belenchia, AM, Beauparlant, P, Mahmood, A, Bajwa, J, Zhang, Q, Khare, S, and Pulakat, L (2017). Cardiovascular Protective vs. Anti-Cancer Properties: Novel Actions of the AT2R Agonist, NP-6A4. The FASEB Journal, 31(1 Supplement), lb680–lb680.
2. Hashimoto, N, Tsunedomi, R, Yoshimura, K, Watanabe, Y, Hazama, S, and Oka, M (2014). Cancer stem-like sphere cells induced from de-differentiated hepatocellular carcinoma-derived cell lines possess the resistance to anti-cancer drugs. BMC Cancer, 14(1), 722.
3. Yallapu, MM, Khan, S, Maher, DM, Ebeling, MC, Sundram, V, Chauhan, N, and Jaggi, M (2014). Anti-cancer activity of curcumin loaded nanoparticles in prostate cancer. Biomaterials, 35(30), 8635–8648.

## EXPERIMENT 8.4

**Aim:** To study the *in vitro* MTT cytotoxicity assays.

**Principle:** The assay can be used for the measurement of cell proliferation in response to growth factors, cytokines, mitogens, nutrients, etc. It can also be used for the analysis of cytotoxic compounds like anticancer drugs and many other toxic agents and pharmaceutical compounds. MTT is used to assess cell viability as a function of redox potential. Actively respiring cells convert the water-soluble MTT to an insoluble purple formazan. The formazan is then solubilized and its concentration determined by optical density.

### Requirements

*Chemicals*: Standard drug solution (vincristine), test sample solution, MTT [3-(4,5-dimethylthiazol-2-yl)-2,5-diphenyltetrazolium bromide] Dulbecco's phosphate-buffered saline (DPBS), dimethylformamide (DMF), sodium dodecyl sulfate (SDS), and glacial acetic acid.

*Equipment*: Microscope.

*Glasswares*: Beakers, pipettes, measuring cylinder, glass rod, slides, and coverslips.

### Procedure

**Reagent preparation MTT solution:**

1. Dissolve MTT in Dulbecco's phosphate buffered saline, pH = 7.4 (DPBS) to 5 mg/mL.
2. Filter-sterilize the MTT solution through a 0.2 μM filter into a sterile, light protected container.
3. Store the MTT solution, protected from light, at 4°C for frequent use or at –20°C for long term storage.

### Solubilization Solution

1. Choose appropriate solvent resistant container and work in a ventilated fume hood. Prepare 40% (vol/vol) dimethylformamide in 2% (vol/vol) glacial acetic acid.
2. Add 16% (wt/vol) sodium dodecyl sulfate (SDS) and dissolve. Adjust to pH = 4.7.
3. Store at room temperature to avoid precipitation of SDS. If a precipitate forms, warm to 37°C and mix to solubilize SDS.

## MTT Assay Protocol

1. Prepare cells and test compounds in 96-well plate containing a final volume of 100 µL/well.
2. Incubate for desired period of exposure.
3. Add 10 µL MTT solution per well to achieve a final concentration of 0.45 mg/mL.
4. Incubate 1–4 hours at 37°C.
5. Add 100 µL solubilization solution to each well to dissolve formazan crystals.
6. Mix to ensure complete solubilization.
7. Record absorbance at 570 nm.

## Observation

| S. no. | Absorbance of control | Absorbance of test | Absorbance of standard |
|--------|-----------------------|--------------------|------------------------|
| 1. | | | |
| 2. | | | |
| 3. | | | |

**Calculation:** The percentage cytotoxic potential is calculated as follows:

$$\text{Percentage cytotoxic potential} = \frac{(\text{Abs control} - \text{Abs sample})}{\text{Abs control}} \times 100$$

where, Abs control—absorbance of control (the control represents 100% viability)

Abs sample—absorbance of sample

## Bibliography

1. Buontempo, F, Orsini, E, Martins, LR, Antunes, I, Lonetti, A, Chiarini, F and Bertaina, A (2014). Cytotoxic activity of the casein kinase 2 inhibitor CX-4945 against T-cell acute lymphoblastic leukemia: targeting the unfolded protein response signaling. Leukemia, 28(3), 543.
2. Kapdi, AR, and Fairlamb, IJ (2014). Anti-cancer palladium complexes: a focus on PdX 2 L 2, palladacycles and related complexes. Chemical Society Reviews, 43(13), 4751–4777.
3. Waseem, D, Butt, AF, Haq, IU, Bhatti, MH, and Khan, GM (2017). Carboxylate derivatives of tributyltin (IV) complexes as anticancer and antileishmanial agents. DARU Journal of Pharmaceutical Sciences, 25(1), 8.

**Aim:** To study the *in vitro* apoptosis by estimation of DNA fragmentation.

**Principle:** Cell and nuclear shrinkage, chromatin condensation, formation of apoptotic bodies and phagocytosis by neighboring cells characterize the main morphological changes of the apoptosis process. Cleavage of chromosomal DNA into oligonucleosomal size fragments is a biochemical hallmark of apoptosis.

## Requirements

*Chemicals*: Standard drug solution (vincristine), test sample solution, 1 N hydrochloric acid solution, acetic acid, alcohol, aceto-orcein or toluidine blue.

*Equipment*: Microscope.

*Glasswares*: Beakers, pipettes, measuring cylinder, glass rod, slides, and coverslips.

## Procedure

**Agarose preparation:**

1. Equilibrate two water baths—one at 40°C and one at ~100°C.
2. Prepare 1% low-gelling-temperature agarose by mixing powdered agarose with distilled water in a glass beaker or bottle.
3. Place bottle in the 100°C water bath for several minutes. Alternatively, carefully microwave bottle at low power for short intervals (avoid vigorous boiling of the agarose and ensure that all agarose is dissolved).
4. Place bottle with agarose into a 40°C water bath. If the cell sample contains red blood cells or hemoglobin, add 2% DMSO to the agarose and/or alkaline lysis solution to avoid damage by iron-catalyzed reactive oxygen species, which can cause strand breaks.

**Slide precoating:**

1. To improve agarose adhesion, score the edges of dust-free frosted-end microscope slides using a diamond-tipped pen.
2. Prepare agarose-precoated slides by dipping the slides into molten 1% agarose and wiping one side clean. It is best to work in a low-humidity environment to ensure agarose adhesion.
3. Allow agarose to air-dry to a thin film. Slides can be prepared ahead of time and stored with desiccant.

**Sample preparation:**

1. Prepare a single-cell suspension using enzyme disaggregation or mechanical dissociation. Never use fixed cells because the DNA will not migrate. Keep cells in ice-cold medium or phosphate-buffered saline to minimize cell aggregation and inhibit DNA repair. Always include a sample of untreated cells to confirm that background damage is low. A positive control [e.g. cells exposed to 20 µM freshly prepared hydrogen peroxide or 8 Gray (Gy) X-rays on ice for the alkaline version, and 75 Gy for the neutral version] is useful when first setting up the method.

2. Using a hemocytometer or particle counter, adjust cell density to about $2 \times 10^4$ cells/mL in phosphate-buffered saline lacking divalent cations.

3. Label slide on frosted end using a pencil, not a pen.

4. Pipet 0.4 mL of cells into a 5 mL plastic disposable tube.

5. Add 1.2 mL 1% low-gelling-temperature agarose at 40°C.

6. Mix and rapidly pipet 1.2 mL of cell suspension onto the agarose-covered surface of a precoated slide; avoid producing bubbles.

7. Allow agarose to gel for about 2 minutes. Be consistent with the time and temperature used for gelling, and ensure that agarose is fully set before submerging in lysis solution.

## Lysis and Electrophoresis

Lysis and electrophoresis can be performed in alkaline (option A) or neutral (option B) conditions. Use option A to detect the combination of DNA single-strand breaks, double-strand breaks and alkali-labile sites in the DNA, and option B to detect only DNA double-strand breaks.

**a. Alkaline lysis and electrophoresis**

i.   After agarose has gelled, submerge slides in a covered dish containing A1 lysis solution. Handle slides gently, e.g. hold slides horizontally and lower into solutions, do not pour solutions over slides or move containers containing slides.

ii.  Lyse samples overnight (18–20 hours) at 4°C in the dark. If time is limited, a 1 hour lysis procedure can also be used, but this will be at the expense of some decrease in sensitivity (up to twofold) and reproducibility.

iii. After 1 hour or overnight lysis, carefully remove slides and submerge in room temperature (18–25°C) A2 rinse solution for 20 minutes. Repeat two times to ensure removal of salt and detergent. Take care not to allow DNA to renature even briefly (i.e. by lowering pH below 12.3) until after electrophoresis, as this will result in DNA tangling and reduced migration.

iv. After these three rinses, submerge slides in fresh A2 solution in an electrophoresis chamber. The chamber should be filled with a consistent volume of buffer that is about 1–2 mm above the top of the agarose.

v. Ensure that the chamber is level using a bubble leveling device. Conduct electrophoresis in solution A2 for 25 minutes at a voltage of 0.6 V/cm. The current should be about 40 mA if using 20 V. The distance in centimeters is measured between the negative and positive electrodes in the electrophoresis chamber.

**b. Neutral lysis and electrophoresis**

i. After agarose has gelled, gently submerge slides in a covered dish containing N1 lysis solution at 4°C, and avoid moving the dish containing the slides.

ii. Place dish in an incubator at 37°C overnight (18–20 hours) in the dark. Although greater sensitivity is achieved using 50°C lysis, the lower temperature reduces heat-labile damage.

iii. After overnight lysis, remove slides and submerge in N2 at room temperature, rinse buffer for 30 minutes at room temperature. Repeat two more times.

iv. Submerge slides in fresh N2 solution in an electrophoresis chamber that has been leveled and filled with a measured volume of buffer about 1–2 mm above the top surface of the agarose.

v. Conduct electrophoresis in solution N2 for 25 minutes at 0.6 V/cm. Current is typically 7 mA when using 20 V.

*Slide Staining*

1. Remove slides from electrophoresis chamber and rinse and neutralize in 400 mL of distilled water.

2. Place slides in staining solution containing 2.5 µg/mL of propidium iodide in distilled water for 20 minutes. Alternatively, pipet 100 µL of a 10 µg/mL stock solution of propidium iodide directly onto the slide and incubate for 20 minutes.

3. Rinse slides with 400 mL distilled water to remove excess stain.

*Slide Analysis*

1. Analyze cells by examining at least 50 comet images from each slide. Avoid analyzing doublets or comets at slide edges. If two or more populations are present, or if heterogeneity in DNA is high, more images should be scored (up to 1,000 can be scored from a slide). When

information on DNA content is required, ensure that the image is not 'saturated', that is, the intensity of fluorescence in any part of the digitized comet image does not exceed the maximum of the digital range (e.g. if 256 channels are available, data should be collected between 0 and 254). This can be accomplished most easily by color-coding the comet image to define specific intensity ranges and then adjusting the light intensity to avoid the color range assigned to channels above 254. Technical methods for extending the dynamic range have also been developed by some comet assay software companies.

2. Using image analysis software, analyze individual comet images for several features including total intensity (DNA content), tail length, percent DNA in tail and tail moment. Alternatively, visual scoring can be used especially when the population is homogenous and noncycling,

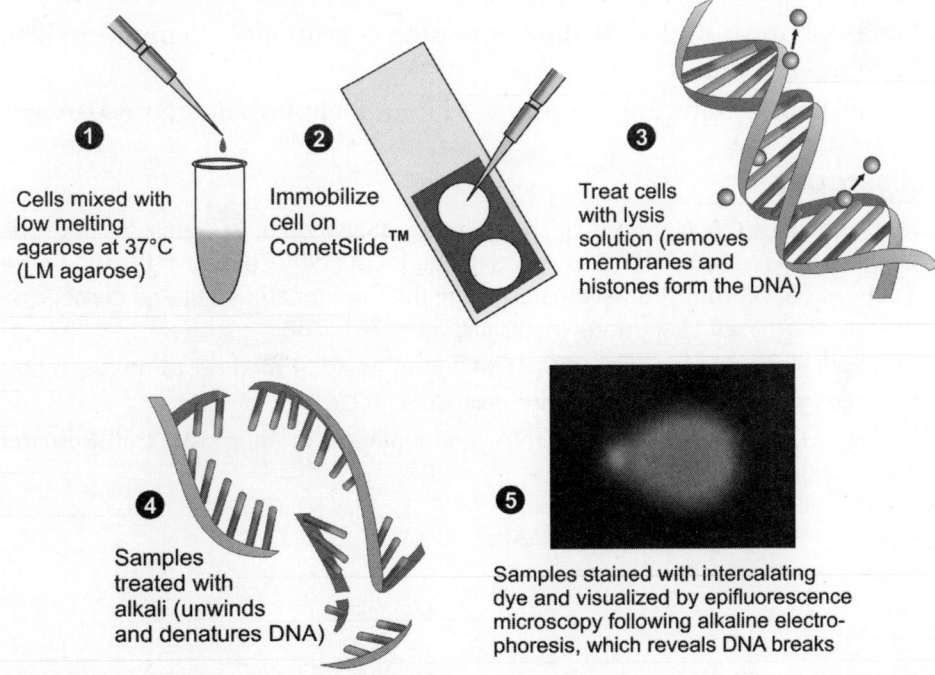

**Fig. 8.4:** Diagrammatic representation of Comet assay procedure and anticipated result

1. Cells are mixed with low-melting point agarose.
2. Immobilised on CometSlide™.
3. Cells are lysed to remove membranes and DNA-associated proteins before alkaline treatment to unwind and denature DNA.
4. During electrophoresis, damaged, unwound, relaxed DNA migrates out of the cell and can be visualized using fluorescent dye (e.g. SYBR® Green).

large differences are expected and adequate controls have been included (e.g. use of coded slides and clearly defined ranges of response). The use of five damage classes introduced by Collins has been widely adopted. Triplicate repeat experiments are recommended.

3. Apply appropriate statistical analysis using means or medians depending on population distributions. Error bars typically represent the between-experiment variability, not the within-slide variability for a specific parameter.

*Timing*

- Slide preparation, cell-sample preparation, agarose embedding for 10 samples—1 hour.
- Alkaline or neutral lysis—typically 18–20 hours, but as short as 1 hour.
- Rinse after lysis—1 hour.
- Electrophoresis under alkaline or neutral conditions—25 minutes. DNA staining—20 minutes.
- Comet image capture and analysis—1 hour for approximately 600 images.

## Bibliography

1. Matzenbacher, CA, Garcia, ALH, dos Santos, MS, Nicolau, CC, Premoli, S, Corrêa, DS, and Kalkreuth, W (2017). DNA damage induced by coal dust, fly and bottom ash from coal combustion evaluated using the micronucleus test and comet assay *in vitro*. Journal of Hazardous Materials, 324, 781–788.
2. Olive, PL, and Banáth, JP (2006). The comet assay: a method to measure DNA damage in individual cells. Nature Protocols, 1(1), 23.
3. Zhang, JH, and Xu, M (2000). DNA fragmentation in apoptosis. Cell Research, 10(3), 205.

## EXPERIMENT 8.6

**Aim:** To study annexin A5-induced apoptosis (annexin A5 affinity assay) by flow cytometery.

**Principle:** Annexin A5 is a member of the annexin protein family that binds in a calcium-dependent way to phosphatidylserine-containing membranes. One of the hallmarks of cell death is the cell surface-expression of phosphatidylserine. Expression of phosphatidylserine at the cell surface can be measured *in vitro* with the phosphatidylserine-binding protein annexin A5 conjugated to fluorochromes. This measurement can be made by flow cytometry or by confocal scanning-laser microscopy. The annexin A5 affinity assay comprises the incubation of cells stimulated to execute cell death with fluorescence-labeled annexin A5 and propidium iodide. Living cells are annexin A5-negative and propidium iodide negative, cells in the early phases of cell death are annexin A5 positive-and propidium iodide-negative, and secondary necrotic cells are annexin A5-positive and propidium iodide-positive. The entire procedure takes about 30 minutes for flow cytometry and 45 minutes for confocal scanning-laser microscopy.

## Requirements

*Chemicals*: Antibody to Fas or other cell death-inducing agents, binding buffer, fixation buffer, green fluorescent annexin A5, propidium iodide, ionomycin, paraformaldehyde, bovine serum albumin, nail polish, and glycerol.

*Equipment*: Flow cytometer and confocal scanning-laser microscope.

*Glasswares*: Beakers, pipettes, measuring cylinder, glass rod, slides, and coverslips.

## Procedure

1. *Method of Reagent Preparation*

   i. *Concentrated binding buffer*: The concentrated binding buffer is 250 mM HEPES plus NaOH, pH 7.4, 1.4 M NaCl, and 10 mM $CaCl_2$. Dilute 10× concentrated binding buffer 1:10 in water for use, to 25 mM HEPES plus NaOH, pH 7.4, 140 mM NaCl, and 1 mM $CaCl_2$. Store binding buffer at 2–8°C. The binding buffer will be stable for 6 months if sterilized by filtration through a filter with a pore size of 2 μm.

   ii. *4% paraformaldehyde fixation buffer*: To prepare 100 mL of 4% (wt/vol) paraformaldehyde fixation buffer, dissolve 4 g paraformaldehyde in 80 mL distilled water. Add some drops of 5 M NaOH and heat the solution to facilitate dissolution of the paraformaldehyde. When the paraformaldehyde is dissolved, add 10 mL of 10× concentrated binding buffer. Adjust the pH to 7.4 with 1 M HCl. Add distilled water to 100 mL.

*Note:* Paraformaldehyde solution must be freshly prepared on the day of use.

## 2. *To Measure PS Expression by Flow Cytometry*

i. Suspend cells at a density of $1 \times 10^6$ cells mL$^{-1}$ in the appropriate medium at 37°C and induce cell death with a selected agent; for example, with 200 ng mL$^{-1}$ antibody to Fas.

ii. As a positive control for cell surface expression of PS, incubate $1 \times 10^6$ cells mL$^{-1}$ with 5 µM ionomycin in binding buffer for 10 minutes. Ionomycin is a calcium ionophore that causes an increase in the intracellular calcium concentration and subsequent expression of PS at the cell surface.

iii. Obtain samples of $5 \times 10^4$ cells (50 µL) at predetermined time points and dilute each sample with 450 µL binding buffer. Add 250 ng mL$^{-1}$ green fluorescent annexin A5 and 250 ng mL$^{-1}$ propidium iodide and incubate the mixture in the dark for 5–15 minutes at 20–25°C (ambient temperature) or on ice, depending on the research question.

iv. Do two-color flow cytometry by binding of green fluorescent annexin A5 at the cell surface. Propidium iodide uptake can be measured without the necessity of including a washing step. If washing steps are required, the wash buffer should contain 1–3 mM CaCl$_2$. The presence of Ca$^{2+}$ ions ensures that the cell-bound annexin A5 remains bound during the washing procedure. The final washing step should also include 250 ng mL$^{-1}$ propidium iodide.

v. Analyze the flow cytometry data 'offline'. Set the quadrants in the green fluorescent annexin A5-versus-propidium iodide dot plot of the untreated control cells. Living cells, annexin A5-binding, and propidium iodide-positive cells are found in the bottom left quadrant, bottom right and top right quadrant, respectively (Fig. 8.5).

## Observation

### Anticipated Result

Figure 8.5 depicts annexin A5 affinity assay by flow cytometry T lymphoma Jurkat cell line using the Jurkat cells were incubated in the absence (Fig. 8.5 A–D) and presence (Fig. 8.5 E–H) of 200 ng mL$^{-1}$ antibody to Fas at

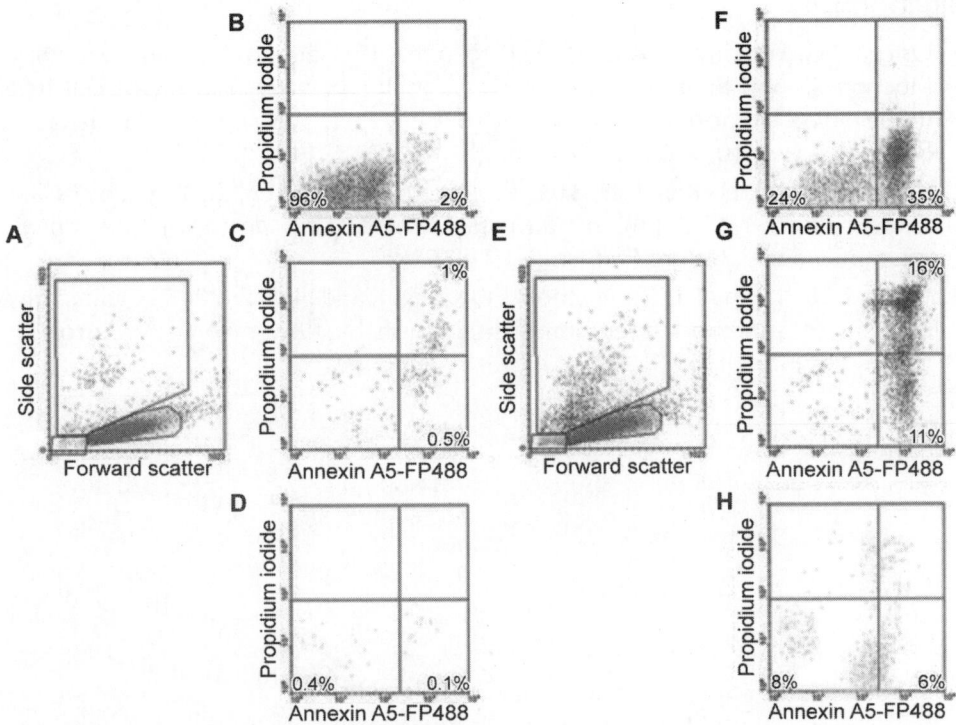

**Fig. 8.5:** Flow cytometry of apoptotic Jurkat cells with annexin A5-FP488 and propidium iodide. Forward- and side-scatter plots of untreated control Jurkat cells (A) and Jurkat cells treated with antibody to Fas (E). (B–D,F–H) Annexin A5-FP488 and propidium iodide dot plots of living and early apoptotic cells (red; B,F), dot plots of dead cells with compromised integrity of the plasma membrane (blue; C,G) and dot plots of apoptotic bodies (green; D,H). Bottom left quadrants, living cells; bottom right quadrants, cells in the early phase of cell death; top right quadrants, cells in the phase of cell death with leaky plasma membrane.

37°C, labeled the cells with annexin A5-FP488 and propidium iodide and then analyzed the cells. Forward-scatter and side-scatter plots of untreated control cells (Fig. 8.5 A) and cells treated with antibody to Fas (Fig. 8.5 E) were obtained. We also obtained annexin A5-FP488- versus propidium iodide dot plots of living and early apoptotic cells (Fig. 8.5 B,F, red), dot plots of dead cells with compromised integrity of the plasma membrane (Fig. 8.5 C, G, blue), and dot plots of apoptotic bodies (Fig. 8.7 D, H, green). Living cells, cells in the early phase of cell death and cells in the phase of cell death with leaky plasma membrane are in the bottom left, bottom right, and top right quadrants, respectively.

## Bibliography

1. Ortega, FG, Fernández-Baldo, MA, Fernández, JG, Serrano, MJ, Sanz, MI, Diaz-Mochón, JJ, and Raba, J (2015). Study of antitumor activity in breast cell lines using silver nanoparticles produced by yeast. International Journal of Nanomedicine, 10, 2021.

2. Van Genderen, H, Kenis, H, Lux, P, Ungeth, L, Maassen, C, Deckers, N and Reutelingsperger, C (2006). *In vitro* measurement of cell death with the annexin A5 affinity assay. Nature Protocols, 1(1), 363.

3. Wang, J, He, L, Chen, D, Pi, Y, Zhou, W, Xiong, X and Hua, Z (2015). Quantitative analysis of annexin V-membrane interaction by flow cytometry. European Biophysics Journal, 44(5), 325–336.

## EXPERIMENT 8.7

**Aim:** To study annexin A5-induced apoptosis (annexin A5 affinity assay) by confocal scanning-laser microscopy (CSLM).

**Principle:** Annexin A5 is a member of the annexin protein family that binds in a calcium-dependent way to phosphatidylserine-containing membranes. One of the hallmarks of cell death is the cell surface-expression of phosphatidylserine. Expression of phosphatidylserine at the cell surface can be measured *in vitro* with the phosphatidylserine-binding protein annexin A5 conjugated to fluorochromes. This measurement can be made by flow cytometry or by confocal scanning-laser microscopy. The annexin A5 affinity assay comprises the incubation of cells stimulated to execute cell death with fluorescence-labeled annexin A5 and propidium iodide. Living cells are annexin A5-negative and propidium iodide negative, cells in the early phases of cell death are annexin A5 positive- and propidium iodide-negative, and secondary necrotic cells are annexin A5-positive and propidium iodide-positive. The entire procedure takes about 30 minutes for flow cytometry and 45 minutes for confocal scanning-laser microscopy.

## Requirements

*Chemicals*: Antibody to Fas or other cell death-inducing agents, binding buffer, fixation buffer, green fluorescent annexin A5, propidium iodide, ionomycin, paraformaldehyde, bovine serum albumin, nail polish, and glycerol.

*Equipment*: Flow cytometer and confocal scanning-laser microscope.

*Glasswares*: Beakers, pipettes, measuring cylinder, glass rod, slides, and coverslips.

## Procedure

*Method of Reagent Preparation*

i. *Concentrated binding buffer*: The concentrated binding buffer is 250 mM HEPES plus NaOH, pH 7.4, 1.4 M NaCl, and 10 mM $CaCl_2$. Dilute 10× concentrated binding buffer 1:10 in water for use, to 25 mM HEPES plus NaOH, pH 7.4, 140 mM NaCl, and 1 mM $CaCl_2$. Store binding buffer at 2–8°C. The binding buffer will be stable for 6 months if sterilized by filtration through a filter with a pore size of 2 μm.

ii. *4% paraformaldehyde fixation buffer*: To prepare 100 mL of 4% (wt/vol) paraformaldehyde fixation buffer, dissolve 4 g paraformaldehyde in 80 mL distilled water. Add some drops of 5 M NaOH and heat the solution to facilitate dissolution of the paraformaldehyde. When the paraformaldehyde is dissolved, add 10 mL of 10× concentrated binding buffer. Adjust the pH to 7.4 with 1 M HCl. Add distilled water to 100 mL.

*Note:* Paraformaldehyde solution must be freshly prepared on the day of use.

## 2. To Measure Phosphatidylserine (PS) Expression by Confocal Scanning-laser Microscopy (CSLM)

i. Suspend cells at a density of $1 \times 10^6$ cells mL$^{-1}$ in the appropriate medium at 37°C and induce cell death with a selected agent. For example, with 200 ng mL$^{-1}$ antibody to Fas.

ii. Add a sample of $5 \times 10^5$ cells mL$^{-1}$ to a microcentrifuge tube and spin cells for 2 minutes at 200 g in a microcentrifuge.

iii. Remove the supernatant and resuspend cells in 500 µL binding buffer. Add 250 ng mL$^{-1}$ of fluorescence labeled annexin A5 and 250 ng mL$^{-1}$ propidium iodide and incubate for 5–15 minutes at ambient temperature or on ice, depending on the research question.

iv. Spin cells in a microcentrifuge for 2 minutes at 200 g and resuspend the cells in 500 µL binding buffer.

v. Spin cells in a microcentrifuge for 2 minutes at 200 g. Remove the supernatant, resuspend cells in 500 µL of 4% paraformaldehyde in binding buffer (the fixation buffer should be freshly prepared) and incubate for 15 minutes at ambient temperature.

*Note:* Cell samples should not be fixed with paraformaldehyde before incubation with fluorescence-labeled annexin A5 because this produces false-positive results. The paraformaldehyde buffer solution should contain $CaCl_2$ at a concentration ranging from 1 mM to 3 mM.

vi. Spin cells in a microcentrifuge for 2 minutes at 200 g. Remove the supernatant and resuspend cells in 500 µL binding buffer supplemented with 1% (wt/vol) bovine serum albumin.

vii. Spin cells in a microcentrifuge for 2 minutes at 200 g. Resuspend cells in 10 µL binding buffer and 30 µL glycerol.

viii. Place 15 µL of the cell suspension on a glass slide and place a glass coverslip over the cell suspension. Seal the glass coverslip onto the glass slide with nail polish and analyze the cells.

## Observation

### Anticipated Result

Cell death was measured with annexin A5 affinity assay by CSLM (Fig. 8.6). Jurkat cells were incubated for 4 hours with 200 ng mL$^{-1}$ antibody to Fas at 37°C, labeled the cells with annexin A5-FP488, green, and propidium iodide, red, and then analyzed them by CSLM. Images of an early apoptotic Jurkat cell (Fig. 8.6 A) and a late apoptotic Jurkat cell with a leaky plasma membrane (Fig. 8.6 B) were obtained.

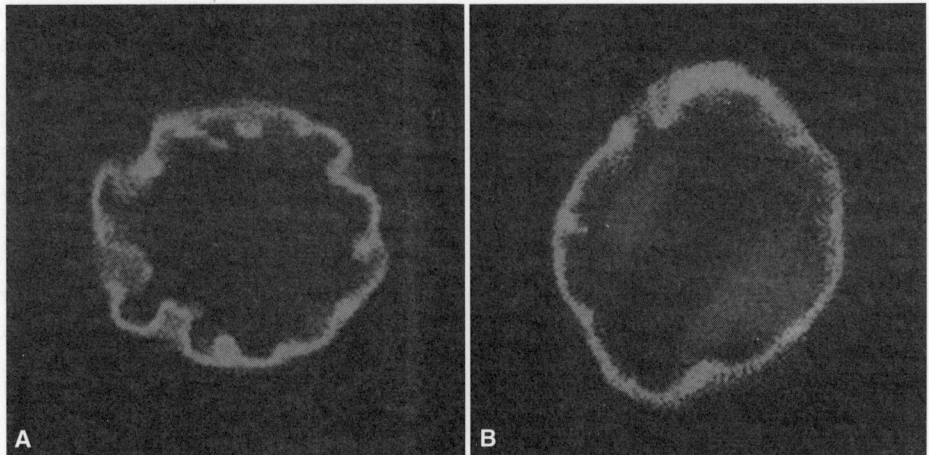

**Fig. 8.6:** CSLM analysis of apoptotic Jurkat cells with annexin A5-FP488 and propidium iodide. Images are of an early apoptotic Jurkat cell (A) and a late apoptotic Jurkat cell with a leaky plasma membrane (B). Original magnification, X63.

## Bibliography

1. Briens, A, Gauberti, M, Parcq, J, Montaner, J, Vivien, D, and de Lizarrondo, SM (2016). Nano-zymography using laser-scanning confocal microscopy unmasks proteolytic activity of cell-derived microparticles. Theranostics, 6(5), 610.

2. Van Genderen, H, Kenis, H, Lux, P, Ungeth, L, Maassen, C, Deckers, N and Reutelingsperger, C (2006). *In vitro* measurement of cell death with the annexin A5 affinity assay. Nature Protocols, 1(1), 363.

## EXPERIMENT 8.8

**Aim:** To study *in vitro* apoptosis by TUNEL assay.

**Principle:** One of the most widely used methods for detecting DNA damage *in situ* is TdT-mediated dUTP-biotin nick end labeling (TUNEL) staining. TUNEL staining was initially described as a method for staining cells that have undergone apoptosis and exhibit internucleosomal DNA fragmentation. TUNEL staining relies on the ability of the enzyme terminal deoxynucleotidyl transferase to incorporate labeled dUTP into free 3'-hydroxyl termini generated by the fragmentation of genomic DNA into low molecular weight double-stranded DNA and high molecular weight single stranded DNA. Cells or tissues are fixed with formaldehyde then permeabilized with ethanol to allow penetration of the TUNEL reaction reagents into the cell nucleus. Following fixation and washing, incorporation of biotinylated dUTP onto the 3' ends of fragmented DNA is carried out in a reaction containing terminal deoxynucleotidyl transferase. The incorporated biotinylated dUTP may be visualized by fluorescence microscopy following staining with fluorescent-tagged avidin or light microscopy following staining with horseradish peroxidase-conjugated avidin-biotin complex in conjunction with a colorimetric substrate.

## Requirements

*Chemicals for cell culture*: Phosphate-buffered saline (PBS), pH 7.4, 2.2% buffered formaldehyde, 70% ethanol, terminal deoxynucleotidyl transferase (TdT) equilibration buffer, Tris-HCl (pH 6.6), potassium cacodylate, $CoCl_2$, bovine serum albumin (BSA). TdT reaction buffer, TdT equilibration buffer, biotinylated-dUTP, TdT staining buffer, saline-sodium citrate, NaCl, sodium citrate, fluorescein isothiocyanate-conjugated avidin, triton X-100, Hoechst 33342 counterstain, Vectashield® antifade mounting medium.

*Chemicals for tissue sections*: Phosphate-buffered saline (PBS), pH 7.4, 4% buffered formaldehyde, proteinase K, ethanol (95, 90, 80, and 70%), 2% hydrogen peroxide, 2% BSA solution, saline sodium citrate (SSC) buffer, NaCl, sodium citrate, TdT equilibration buffer, 2.5 mM Tris-HCl (pH 6.6), 0.2 M potassium cacodylate, 2.5 mM $CoCl_2$, BSA, TdT reaction buffer, TdT enzyme, biotinylated-dUTP, Vectastain ABC-peroxidase stock solution, 3,3'-diaminobenzidine (DAB) staining solution, TdT staining buffer, 2.5 µg/mL fluorescein isothiocyanate-conjugated avidin, 0.1% triton X-100, and 1% BSA, hematoxylin counterstain, hoechst 33342 counterstain, Vectashield® antifade mounting medium.

*Equipment*: V-bottomed 96-well plate, fluorescence microscope and light microscope.

*Glasswares*: Beakers, pipettes, measuring cylinder, glass rod, slides and coverslips.

## Procedure

1. *Method of reagent preparation*

**Reagents for cell culture**

   i. 2% buffered formaldehyde—dilute high quality formaldehyde (v/v) in PBS prior to use

   ii. TdT equilibration buffer: 2.5 mM Tris-HCl (pH 6.6), 0.2 M potassium cacodylate, 2.5 mM $CoCl_2$, 0.25 mg/mL bovine serum albumin (BSA). Aliquots may be stored at –20°C for several months.

   iii. TdT reaction buffer—TdT equilibration buffer containing 0.5 U/µL of TdT enzyme and 40 pmol/µL biotinylated-dUTP. Prepare fresh from stock solutions prior to use.

   iv. TdT staining buffer—4× saline-sodium citrate (0.6 M NaCl, 60 mM sodium citrate)

   v. 1% BSA—prepare fresh from stock solutions prior to use

   vi. Hoechst 33342 counterstain—2 µg/mL in PBS. Stock solution may be stored at 4°C in the dark for several weeks.

**Reagents for cell culture**

   i. 4% buffered formaldehyde—dilute high quality formaldehyde (v/v) in PBS prior to use

   ii. 20 µg/mL proteinase K, stock solution may be stored at –20°C for several months.

   iii. 2% hydrogen peroxide—prepare fresh from hydrogen peroxide reagent stock prior to use

   iv. 2% BSA solution—2% BSA (w/v) dissolved in PBS and passed through a 0.45 µm filter. Sterile stock solution may be stored at 4°C for several weeks.

   v. SSC buffer—300 mM NaCl, 30 mM sodium citrate. Stock solution may be stored at room temperature for several months.

   vi. TdT equilibration buffer—2.5 mM Tris-HCl (pH 6.6), 0.2 M potassium cacodylate, 2.5 mM $CoCl_2$, 0.25 mg/mL BSA. Prepare from stock solutions. Aliquots may be stored at –20°C for several months.

vii. TdT reaction buffer—TdT equilibration buffer containing 0.5 U/µL of TdT enzyme and 40 pmol/µL biotinylated-dUTP. Prepare fresh from stock solutions prior to use.

viii. TdT staining buffer—4× saline-sodium citrate (0.6 M NaCl, 60 mM sodium citrate)

ix. Hoechst 33342 counterstain—2 µg/mL in PBS (molecular probes). Stock solution may be stored at 4°C in the dark for several weeks.

## 2. *TUNEL Assay for Cell Suspension*

i. Collect cells by centrifugation, wash with PBS, and resuspend cells at a concentration of $1–2 \times 10^7$ cells/mL in PBS. Transfer 100 µL of cell suspension to a V-bottomed 96-well plate.

ii. Fix cells by addition of 100 µL of 2% formaldehyde in PBS, pH 7.4.

iii. Incubate on ice for 15 minutes.

iv. Collect cells by centrifugation, wash once with 200 µL PBS, the postfix with 200 µL of 70% ice-cold ethanol. Cells may be stored in 70% ethanol at –20°C for several days.

v. Collect cells by centrifugation and wash twice with 200 µL PBS.

vi. Resuspend cells ($1 \times 10^5–5 \times 10^5$ cells/mL) in 50 µL of TdT equilibration buffer. Incubate the cell suspension at 37°C for 10 minutes with occasional gentle mixing.

vii. Resuspend cells in 50 µL of TdT reaction buffer. Incubate the cell suspension at 37°C for 30 minutes with occasional gentle mixing.

viii. Collect cells by centrifugation and wash with 200 µL PBS.

ix. Resuspend the cells in 100 µL of TdT staining buffer. Incubate the cell suspension at room temperature for 30 minutes in the dark.

x. Collect cells by centrifugation, wash twice with 200 µL PBS, then resuspend in PBS at $2–8 \times 10^6$ cells/mL. For fluorescence microscopy attach coverslips using Vectashield® antifade mounting medium.

xi. Examine cells by fluorescence microscopy, confocal microscopy or flow cytometry.

## 3. *TUNEL assay for Cytospin Cell Suspension*

i. Collect cells by centrifugation, wash with PBS, then collect on glass slides pretreated with aqueous 0.01% poly-L-lysine using a cytospin device. Routinely $1 \times 10^5 – 5 \times 10^5$ cells/mL are collected on a single slide.

ii. Fix cells by covering with a puddle of 1% formaldehyde in PBS for 15 minutes.

iii. Rinse slides with PBS then transfer to a Coplin jar containing ice-cold 70% ethanol for 1 hour. Slides may be stored overnight in 70% ethanol at 4°C.

iv. Rinse slides with PBS and pipet 25–50 µL of TdT buffer onto the slides, enough to cover the cells. Incubate the slides in a humidified chamber for 30 minutes at 37°C. In order to conserve reagents a reduced volume of TdT buffer may be used and carefully covered with a glass coverslip during the incubation. Take care to avoid trapping air bubbles which may lead to staining artifacts.

v. Rinse the slides with PBS then pipet 25–50 µL of TdT staining buffer onto the slides. Incubate for 30 minutes at room temperature in the dark.

vi. Rinse the slides with PBS, air dry, and attach coverslips using Vectashield® antifade mounting medium.

vii. Examine cells by fluorescence or confocal microscopy.

4. *TUNEL Assay for Tissue Section by Colorimetric Staining for Light Microscopy*

i. Fix tissue samples in 4% formaldehyde in PBS for 24 hours and embed in paraffin.

ii. Adhere 4–6 µm paraffin sections to glass slides pretreated with 0.01% aqueous solution of poly-L-lysine.

iii. Deparaffinize sections by heating the slides for 30 minutes at 60°C (or 10 minutes at 70°C) followed by two 5 minutes incubations in a xylene bath at room temperature in Coplin jars. Rehydrate the tissue samples by transferring the slides through a graded ethanol series—2 × 3 minutes 96% ethanol, 1 × 3 minutes 90% ethanol, 1 × 3 minutes 80% ethanol, 1 × 3 minutes 70% ethanol, 1 × 3 minutes double-distilled water (DDW).

iv. Carefully blot away excess water and pipet 20 µg/mL proteinase K solution to cover sections. Incubate 15 minutes at room temperature.

v. Following proteinase K treatment, wash slides 3 × 5 minutes with DDW. Inactivate endogenous peroxidases by covering sections with 2% hydrogen peroxide for 5 minutes at room temperature. Wash slides 3 × 5 minutes with DDW.

vi. Carefully blot away excess water then cover sections with TdT equilibration buffer for 10 minutes at room temperature.

vii. Remove TdT equilibration buffer and cover sections with TdT reaction buffer.

viii. Incubate slides in a humidified chamber for 30 minutes at 37°C. In order to conserve reagents a reduced volume of TdT buffer may be carefully covered with a glass coverslip during the incubation. Take care to avoid trapping air bubbles which may lead to staining artifacts.

ix.   Stop reaction by incubating slides 2 × 10 minutes in 2 × SSC.

x.   Rinse slides in PBS then block nonspecific binding by covering tissue sections with 2% BSA solution for 30–60 minutes at room temperature.

xi.   Wash slides 2 × 5 minutes in PBS then incubate in Vectastain ABC-peroxidase solution for 1 hour at 37°C.

xii.   Wash slides 2 × 5 minutes in PBS then stain with DAB staining solution at room temperature. Monitor color development until desired level of staining is achieved (typically 10–60 minutes). Stop the reaction by incubating slides in DDW.

xiii.   Lightly counterstain tissue sections with hematoxylin stain.

xiv.   Cover tissue sections with coverslips using aqua-poly/mount mounting medium.

xv.   Observe sections under light microscopy.

### 5. *TUNEL Assay for Tissue Section by Fluorescent Staining*

i.   Fix tissue samples in 4% formaldehyde in PBS for 24 hours and embed in paraffin.

ii.   Adhere 4–6 μm paraffin sections to glass slides pretreated with 0.01% aqueous solution of poly-L-lysine.

iii.   Deparaffinize sections by heating the slides for 30 minutes at 60°C (or 10 minutes at 70°C) followed by two 5 minutes incubations in a xylene bath at room temperature in Coplin jars. Rehydrate the tissue samples by transferring the slides through a graded ethanol series—2 × 3 minutes 96% ethanol, 1 × 3 minutes 90% ethanol, 1 × 3 minutes 80% ethanol, 1 × 3 minutes 70% ethanol, 1 × 3 minutes double-distilled water (DDW).

iv.   Carefully blot away excess water and pipet 20 μg/mL proteinase K solution to cover sections. Incubate for 15 minutes at room temperature.

v.   Following proteinase K treatment, wash slides 3 × 5 minutes with DDW.

vi.   Carefully blot away excess water then cover sections with TdT equilibration buffer for 10 minutes at room temperature.

vii.   Remove TdT equilibration buffer and cover sections with TdT reaction buffer.

viii.   Incubate slides in a humidified chamber for 30 minutes at 37°C. In order to conserve reagents a reduced volume of TdT buffer may be carefully covered with a glass coverslip during the incubation. Take care to avoid trapping air bubbles which may lead to staining artifacts.

ix.   Stop reaction by incubating slides 2 × 10 minutes in 2 ×SSC.

x. Wash slides 2 × 5 minutes in PBS then cover tissue sections with TdT staining buffer. Incubate slides at room temperature for 30 minutes in the dark.

xi. Wash slides 2 × 5 minutes in PBS.

xii. Lightly counterstain sections with hematoxylin, Hoechst 33342 or other appropriate counterstain.

xiii. Wash slides with PBS, air dry, and attach coverslips using Vectashield® antifade mounting medium.

xiv. Examine tissue sections by fluorescence or confocal microscopy.

## 6. TUNEL Assay for DNA Strand Break Labeling with Br-dUTP for Analysis by Flow Cytometry

i. Suspend $1-2 \times 10^6$ cells/mL in 0.5 mL PBS. Transfer this suspension with a Pasteur pipette into a 5 mL polypropylene tube containing 4.5 mL of ice cold 1% formaldehyde in PBS. Keep the tube for 15 minutes on ice.

ii. Centrifuge at 300 g for 5 minutes, resuspend cell pellet in 5 mL of PBS, centrifuge again and resuspend cell pellet in 0.5 mL of PBS. With a Pasteur pipette transfer the suspension to a tube containing 4.5 mL of ice-cold 70% ethanol. The cells can be stored in ethanol for several weeks at 20°C.

iii. Centrifuge at 200 g for 3 minutes, remove ethanol, resuspend cells in 5 mL of PBS and centrifuge again at 300 g for 5 minutes.

iv. Resuspend the pellet in 50 µl of a solution containing:
   - 10 µL TdT 5· reaction buffer.
   - 2.0 µL of Br-dUTP stock solution.
   - 0.5 µL (12.5 U) TdT.
   - 5 µL $CoCl_2$ solution.
   - 33.5 µL distilled $H_2O$.

v. Incubate the cells in this solution for 40 minutes at 37°C.

vi. Add 1.5 mL of the rinsing buffer, and centrifuge at 300 g for 5 minutes).

vii. Resuspend cell pellet in 100 µl of FITC-conjugated anti-BrdU mAb solution.

viii. Incubate at room temperature for 1 hour.

ix. Add 1 mL of PI staining solution.

x. Incubate for 30 minutes at room temperature, or 20 minutes at 37°C, in the dark.

xi. Analyze cells by flow cytometry.
   - Excite fluorescence with blue light (488 nm laser line or BG12 excitation filter).

- Measure green fluorescence of FITC- anti-Br-dUAb at 530 ±20 nm.
- Measure red fluorescence of PI at >600 nm.

## Observation and Anticipated Result

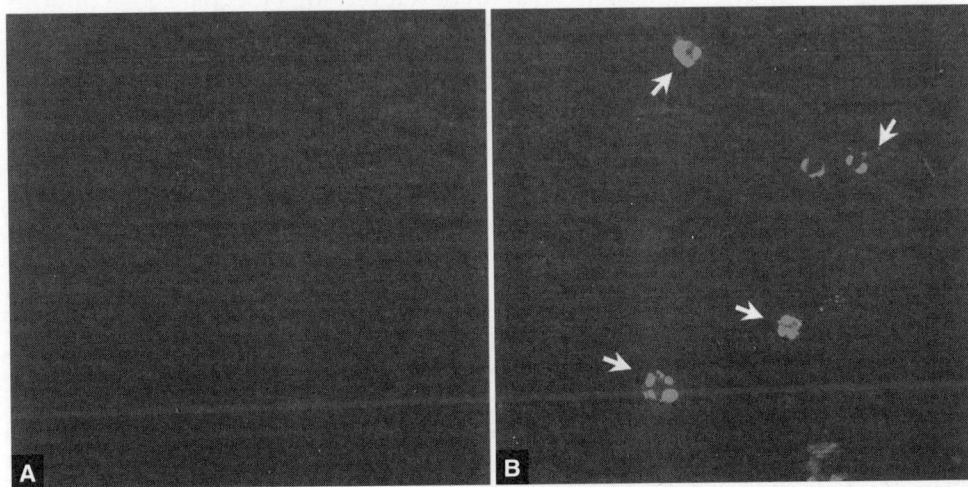

**Fig. 8.7:** Confocal micrograph of TUNEL-stained Jurkat T lymphocytes. (A) Untreated culture. (B) Fas ligand-treated culture undergoing apoptosis.
*Note*: Arrows in (B) point towards the condensed TUNEL-positive chromatin within the nuclei of cells undergoing apoptosis.

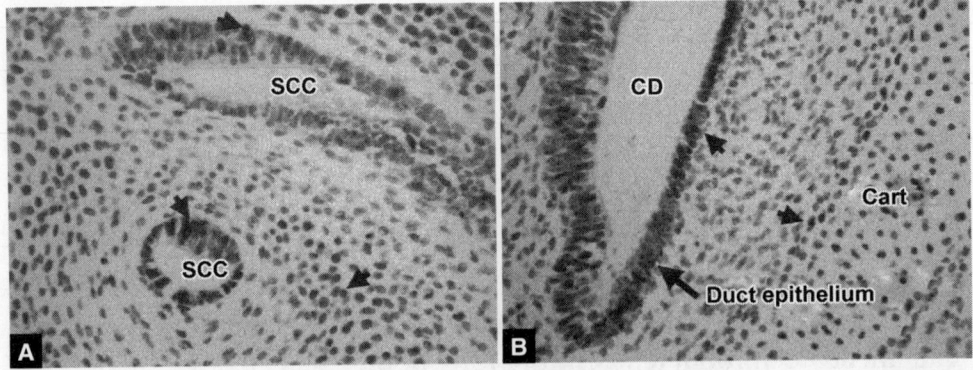

**Fig. 8.8A and B:** Micrographs of TUNEL-stained mouse embryo tissue undergoing developmental restructuring (E11-12). (A) Semicircular canal area. (B) Cochlear duct and primordial cartilage. Apoptotic cells within the duct epithelium and adjacent primordial cartilage exhibiting DNA damage are stained brown (see arrowheads). Sections are counterstained with hematoxylin (blue staining) to identify background TUNEL-negative cells and associated morphology.

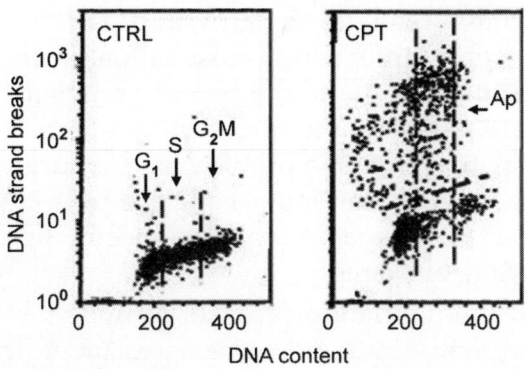

**Fig. 8.9:** Scatterplots illustrating the detection of DNA strand breaks in apoptotic cells by TUNEL assay. HL-60 cells were untreated (CTRL) or treated with 200 nM DNA topoisomerase 1 inhibitor camptothecin (CPT) for 3 hours, fixed and processed according to the prescribed protocol. Cellular DNA was stained with PI while DNA strand breaks were labeled with Br-dUTP followed by the FITC-conjugated Br-dUAb. Based on the differences in DNA content one can identify cells in G1 vs S vs G2M phases of the cell cycle as shown in the left panel (separated by the dashed vertical boundaries). Apoptotic cells (Ap) are characterized by very high frequency of DNA strand breaks (note exponential scale of Y coordinate). It is quite evident that CPT-induced apoptosis preferentially of S-phase cells.

## Bibliography

1. Darzynkiewicz, Z, Galkowski, D, and Zhao, H (2008). Analysis of apoptosis by cytometry using TUNEL assay. Methods, 44(3), 250–254.
2. Loo DT (2002). Tunel Assay. In: Didenko V.V. (eds) In Situ Detection of DNA Damage. Methods in Molecular Biology, vol 203. Humana Press.

## *IN VITRO* ANGIOGENESIS

Angiogenesis is the growth of blood vessels from the existing vasculature. It occurs throughout life in both health and disease, beginning *in utero* and continuing on through old age. No metabolically active tissue in the body is more than a few hundred micrometers from a blood capillary, which is formed by the process of angiogenesis. Capillaries are needed in all tissues for diffusion exchange of nutrients and metabolites. Changes in metabolic activity lead to proportional changes in angiogenesis and, hence, proportional changes in capillarity. Oxygen plays a pivotal role in this regulation. Hemodynamic factors are critical for survival of vascular networks and for structural adaptations of vessel walls.

Tumor angiogenesis refers to the growth of new vessels toward and within the tumor; unless tumor neovascularization occurs, cell proliferation reaches a steady state, and the tumor grows no larger than about 2 mm greatest diameter. Moreover, for tumor cells to metastasize, they must gain access to the vasculature from the primary tumor, survive the circulation, localize in the target organ, and induce angiogenesis in that target organ. Tumor angiogenesis is necessary both at the beginning and at the end of the metastatic cascade of events.

Angiogenesis is an important process for forming new blood vessels. It is fundamental in many biological processes including development, reproduction, and wound repair. Under these conditions, angiogenesis is a highly regulated process. Numerous inducers of angiogenesis have been identified, including the members of the vascular endothelial growth factor family, angiopoietins, transforming growth factors, platelet-derived growth factor, tumor necrosis factor-$\alpha$, interleukins and members of the fibroblast growth factor family. Vascular endothelial growth factor-A is the most potent proangiogenic protein described to date. It induces proliferation, sprouting and tube formation of endothelial cells. Angiogenesis is therefore a putative target for therapy. The potential application of different angiogenesis inhibitors is currently under intense clinical investigation.

## Factors in Regulating Angiogenesis

**Vascular endothelial growth factor:** Vascular endothelial growth factor-A (VEGF-A; also referred to as VEGF) is the best characterized and the most studied of the VEGF family members. It is a tumor-secreted cytokine with grave importance in both normal and tumor associated angiogenesis. VEGF-A exerts its biologic effect through interaction with cell surface receptors. These receptors are transmembrane tyrosine kinase receptors and they include VEGF receptor-1 (VEGFR-1) and VEGFR-2, selectively expressed on vascular endothelial cells, and the neuropilin receptors (NP-1 and NP-2), expressed on neurons and vascular endothelium. VEGF-A is the most potent proangiogenic protein described to date. It induces proliferation, sprouting and tube formation of endothelial cells. In addition, it causes vasodilatation by inducing the endothelial nitric oxide synthase and so increasing nitric oxide production.

**Angiopoietins and tie receptors:** Another signaling system involved in vessel maintenance, growth and stabilization is the Tie2 receptor, which binds the angiopoietins (Ang1 and Ang2). The four identified angiopoietins are a family of secreted proteins that bind Tie receptors. Angiopoietins and Tie receptors play a key role in angiogenesis. Expression patterns of the two Tie receptors, Tie1 and Tie2, are similar to those of VEGFRs. Tie1 mRNA is highly expressed in embryonic vascular endothelium, angioblasts, and endocardium, whereas it is expressed strongly in lung capillaries but weakly in endocardium in adult tissues.

**Fibroblast growth factor:** Acidic and basic fibroblast growth factors (aFGF and bFGF, respectively) are heparin-binding protein mitogens that are thought to play an important role in angiogenesis. aFGF was the first factor of the family to be associated with angiogenesis. *In vitro*, both aFGF and bFGF induce many processes in the endothelial cells that are significant to angiogenesis.

**Platelet-derived growth factor (PDGF)** was initially purified from platelets and was then identified in fibroblasts, astrocytes, keratinocytes, epithelial cells and other cell types. PDGFs exist as heterodimers (PDGF-AB) or homodimers (PDGF-AA or -BB) composed of chains A and B. PDGF receptors are made up of complexes between α and β subtypes. Although implicated, the role of PDGF in angiogenesis is not yet fully understood whereas the FGF and VEGF have attracted more interest as possible therapeutic targets.

**Transforming growth factor-β:** The transforming growth factor-βs (TGF-β) represent a family of highly conserved cytokines typified by TGF-β1. Both pro- and antiangiogenic properties have been ascribed to TGF-β1, through effects on endothelial cells and other cell types.

## Membrane-bound Factors Important in Angiogenesis

A number of membrane-bound proteins play important roles in angiogenesis. Integrins, ephrins, and cadherins are membrane-bound proteins that affect many functions involved in blood vessel assembly. In particular, αvβ3-integrin, ephrin-2B, and VE-cadherin affect the process of angiogenesis.

## Role of the Plasminogen Activator/Plasmin System in Angiogenesis

Plasmin is a broad-spectrum protease which is presumed to hydrolyze many extracellular proteins, most notably fibrin. Urokinase-type plasminogen activator (uPA) and tissue plasminogen activator (tPA) are serine proteases that mainly activate plasminogen; plasminogen is their specific substrate. uPA is a serine protease that binds to a specific glycosylphosphatidylinositol-anchored cell surface receptor (uPA receptor-uPAR). Assessing the role of the individual components of the PA/plasmin system in angiogenesis *in vivo* was made possible by the generation of mice deficient in these components. Plasminogen activator inhibitor type-1 (PAI-1) is considered one of the key regulators of tumor invasion, metastasis, as well as cancer-related angiogenesis.

### Role of Hypoxia-inducible Factor in Angiogenesis

Hypoxia-inducible factor-1 (HIF-1) is an αβ-heterodimer that was first recognized as a DNA-binding factor that mediates hypoxia-inducible activity of the erythropoietin 3′ enhancer. Following this, it rapidly became clear that the HIF system is a key regulator of many other processes among which is angiogenesis. Consistent with a major role for hypoxia in the overall process of angiogenesis, a large number of genes involved in different steps of angiogenesis are independently responsive to hypoxia in tissue culture. Examples include nitric oxide synthasis involved in governing vascular tone, growth factors such as VEGF, angiopoietins, fibroblast growth factors, and their various receptors, and genes involved in matrix metabolism, including matrix metalloproteinases, plasminogen activator receptors and inhibitors, and collagen prolyl hydroxylase.

Angiogenesis is a complex and important process in a variety of physiological processes including embryonic development, ovulation, wound repair, and collateral vessel formation in the myocardium. The recognition that angiogenesis plays a critical role in a variety of pathologic conditions, including tumor growth, led to the discovery of several pro- and antiangiogenic factors and strategies. Angiogenesis is therefore a putative target for therapy. The potential application of different angiogenesis inhibitors is currently under intense clinical investigation. A better understanding of the biology of angiogenesis may reveal new targets for treating many diseases that are associated with this complex process.

## Bibliography

1. Otrock, ZK, Mahfouz, RA, Makarem, JA, and Shamseddine, AI (2007). Understanding the biology of angiogenesis: review of the most important molecular mechanisms. Blood Cells, Molecules, and Diseases, 39(2), 212–220.

2. Shahi, PK, and Pineda, IF (2008). Tumoral angiogenesis: review of the literature. Cancer Investigation, 26(1), 104–108.

3. Yadav, L, Puri, N, Rastogi, V, Satpute, P, and Sharma, V (2015). Tumour angiogenesis and angiogenic inhibitors: A review. Journal of clinical and diagnostic research: JCDR, 9(6), XE01.

**Aim:** To study the antiangiogenic activity of the given sample by chorioallantoic membrane assay (CAM).

**Principle:** Chorioallantoic membrane assay is performed by implanting a membrane or coverslip containing the compound of interest on the chick embryo chorioallantoic membrane. During avian development the mesodermal layers of the allantois and chorion fuse to form the chorioallantoic membrane. This structure rapidly expands generating a rich vascular network that provides an interface for gas and waste exchange. The CAM allows to study tissue grafts, tumor growth and metastasis, drugs delivery and toxicologic analysis, and angiogenic and antiangiogenic molecules. The CAM is relatively simple, quick, and low-cost model that allows screening of a large number of pharmacological samples. Antiangiogenic potential of the sample can be quantified via image analysis or colorimetric detection methods.

## Requirements

*Chemicals*: Benzalkonium bromide, 0.9% isotonic saline, sample drug, and reference standard.

*Equipment*: Incubator.

*Glasswares*: Beakers, pipettes, measuring cylinder, glass rod, slides, and coverslips.

## Procedure

1. Clean fertilized chicken embryos (48 ± 5 g) with 0.1% benzalkonium bromide and preincubated at 37.5°C in 85% humidity for 2 days.
2. Egg morphology appears like a metaellipse, with a relatively larger side and a smaller one, and the air sac is usually located on the larger side right behind the shell. After disinfection of the shell center outside the air sac with 0.1% benzalkonium bromide, buff, and gently drill a hole highlighted with marker pen over the air sac with a nipper not to break the shell, and the vascular zone is easy to be identified on the CAM (Fig. 8.10).
3. Two drops of normal saline is added to moisten the inner shell membrane adjacent to the CAM so that the membrane was easy to be separated from CAM.
4. After being clamped and raised by ophthalmic forceps, the membrane and the CAM separated unforcedly, and section a 1 × 1 cm window on the membrane to expose the vascular zone.

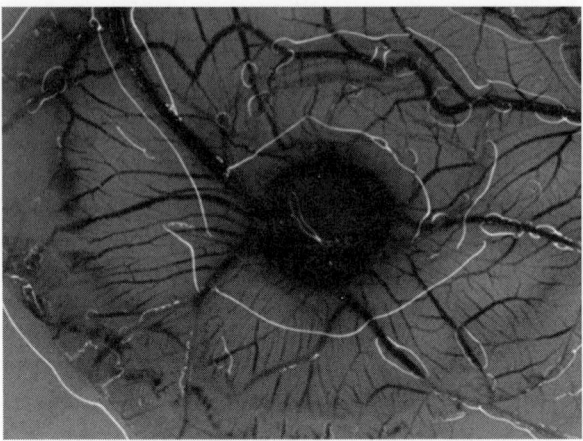

**Fig. 8.10:** The vascular zone of the CAM

5. A 5 mm × 5 mm sterilized filter-paper disks, used as a carrier for directly loading the indicated concentrations of sample drug, is then directly applied and adhered to the vascular zone.

6. Seal the openings with sterile flexible packing film, and further incubate the eggs for indicated periods for 1–3 days depending on the compound under study.

7. Finally mix methanol and acetone (1:1 in volume) and add directly to immerse and fix the blood vessels of the experiment zone.

8. Clamp and raise the CAM by ophthalmic forceps to separate it from the embryo, and cut to spread on glass slide. The blood vessels can be viewed, photographed or quantified by counting the number of blood vessel branch points (Fig. 8.11).

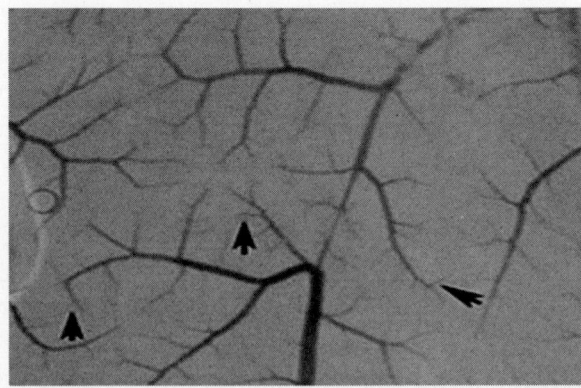

**Fig. 8.11:** Blood vessel branch points on CAM (arrows indicate new-formed blood vessel branches)

## Observation

| S. no. | Number of blood vessel branching points | | |
| --- | --- | --- | --- |
| | Control | Test | Standard |
| 1. | | | |
| 2. | | | |
| 3. | | | |

**Calculation:** The percentage inhibition of angiogenesis is calculated as follows:

Percentage antiangiogenesis = $[(N_C–N_T)/ L_C]100$

where, $N_C$—number of blood vessel branching points in control group

$N_T$—number of blood vessel branching points in test group

## Bibliography

1. Chen, Z, Wen, Z and Bai, X (2013). In vivo Chick Chorioallantoic Membrane (CAM) Angiogenesis Assays. Bio-protocol 3(18): e913.

2. Chen, Z, Zhang, Y, Jia, C, Wang, Y, Lai, P, Zhou, X, Wang, Y, Song, Q, Lin, J, Ren, Z, Gao, Q, Zhao, Z, Zheng, H, Wan, Z, Gao, T, Zhao, A, Dai, Y and Bai, X (2014). mTORC1/2 targeted by n-3 polyunsaturated fatty acids in the prevention of mammary tumorigenesis and tumor progression. Oncogene, 33(37): 4548–4557.

3. Wen, ZH, Su, YC, Lai, PL, Zhang, Y, Xu, YF, Zhao, A, Yao, GY, Jia, CH, Lin, J, Xu, S, Wang, L, Wang, XK, Liu, AL, Jiang, Y, Dai, YF and Bai, XC (2013). Critical role of arachidonic acid-activated mTOR signaling in breast carcinogenesis and angiogenesis. Oncogene, 32(2): 160–170.

## EXPERIMENT 8.10

**Aim:** To study the antiangiogenic activity of the given sample by endothelial cell tube formation assay.

**Principle:** The *in vitro* formation of capillary-like tubes by endothelial cells on a basement membrane matrix is a powerful *in vitro* method to screen for various factors that promote or inhibit angiogenesis. The protocol presented here is for rapid, quantitative, and reliable *in vitro* angiogenesis assay that can be adapted for high throughput use. Endothelial cells are plated on a gelled basement matrix to form capillary-like structures with a lumen. The assay can be used to identify inhibitors or stimulators of angiogenesis, as well as genes and signaling pathways involved in angiogenesis. It has also been used to identify endothelial progenitor cells. This assay involves endothelial cell adhesion, migration, protease activity and tubule formation. This tube formation assay is preferred, as other *in vitro* assays for angiogenesis, such as cell adhesion, migration and invasion as they measure limited steps in the angiogenesis process. Additionally the assay has the advantage of completing in a day as transformed endothelial cells form tubes within 3 hours, whereas nontransformed endothelial cells form tubes within 6 hours.

### Requirements

*Chemicals*: Basement membrane extract, reduced growth factor, human umbilical vein endothelial cells (HUVECs), trypsin-EDTA, phosphate-buffered saline, 0.4% (w/v) trypan blue solution, endothelial cell growth medium-2 (EGM-2) single quot kit, endothelial basal medium-2 (EBM-2), recombinant human FGF basic (basic fibroblast growth factor, bFGF), sulforaphane, dimethyl sulfoxide (DMSO), phosphate-buffered saline, calcein AM, cell staining solution, and methanol.

*Equipment*: Cell culture incubator (humidified, 5% $CO_2$), biological hood with laminar flow and UV light, water bath, centrifuge with a swing-bucket rotor, hemocytometer, inverted phase microscope with fluorescence.

*Glasswares*: 96-well cell culture plates, 15 mL conical centrifuge tubes-sterile, Tissue culture flasks, 25 $cm^2$, filter cap, 50 mL disposable sterile plastic pipettes, pipette aid, and sterile micropipette.

### Procedure

1. *Method of Preparation of Reagents*

   i. Endothelial cell growth medium-2: Add all supplements and growth factors of the EGM-2 to EBM-2 and store at 4°C for up to 1 month.

ii. bFGF stock solution: Make a 10 mM stock of bFGF in sterile PBS with 0.1% (vol/vol) bovine serum albumin, aliquot, and store at –20°C for up to 6 months.

iii. 10 mM sulforaphane: Make a 10 mM stock of sulforaphane in DMSO solution and store at 4°C for up to 1 month. For long-term storage, aliquot and store at –20°C for up to 6 months.

iv. 2 mM calcein AM stock solution: Dissolve lyophilized calcein AM in DMSO solution and keep at 4°C for up to 1 month. For long-term storage, aliquot and store at –20°C for up to 6 months.

## 2. Passaging of Human Umbilical Vein Endothelial Cells

- *Time duration*: 30 minutes (1 day before assay start)

  Using standard procedures to passage cells, split nearly confluent flasks of HUVECs such that cells will be ~80% confluent in 24 hours. Generally, plating $5 \times 10^5$ to $1 \times 10^6$ cells/mL in a 25 cm$^2$ flask works well.

## 3. Thaw the Basement Membrane Extract

- *Time duration*: 5 minutes (1 day before assay start)

  Remove the basement membrane extract from the –20°C or –80°C freezer and place in a refrigerator at 4°C.

**Note:** The basement membrane extract gels very easily, hence it is important not to warm it as part of the thawing process and to keep it on ice while pipetting in the cell culture plates. It may be aliquoted and frozen at –20°C or –80°C; or stored at 4°C for a few days. Before aliquoting, invert a tube with basement membrane extract a few times.

## 4. Coating 96-well Cell Culture Plate with Basement Membrane Extract

- *Time duration*: 10–20 minutes
  i. Label wells (in triplicate) of 96-well plate as follows: 35 nm mL 1 bFGF with 10 mM bFGF. Place a tube of fully thawed basement membrane extract and labeled 96-well plate on ice in a laminar flow hood. Invert the tube with extract a few times to mix the contents. Load 50–80 µL of the basement membrane extract per well of 96-well plate.

**Note:** Avoid air bubbles in the basement membrane extract by carefully pipetting the liquid into wells. If air bubbles get trapped in the wells, centrifuge the plate at $300 \times g$ for 10 minutes at 4°C. Make sure that centrifuge is precooled to 4°C before placing a plate with basement membrane extract in it.

ii. Transfer 96-well plate to a cell culture incubator and incubate it at 37°C for 30 minutes to allow the basement membrane to gel.

**Note:** Do not shake the plate during gelling time as this will result in an uneven surface on the gel.

### 5. *Harvest 80% Confluent HUVECs from 25 cm² Flask*

- *Time duration*: 10 minutes
  i. Warm PBS, trypsin-EDTA, EGM-2 and EBM-2 in the 37°C water bath.
  ii. Remove and discard the media from 25 cm² flask with HUVECs and rinse cells with PBS. Add 1 mL of trypsin-EDTA to the flask, swirl briefly and incubate at 37°C for a few minutes to release the cells. Tap the side of the flask to be sure that the cells are detaching.

### 6. *Quantitate and Collect Cells*

- *Time duration*: 15 minutes
  i. Add 1 mL of growth medium EGM-2; gently pipette the solution up and down to make a single cell suspension. Transfer cell suspension in a sterile 15 mL conical tube.
  ii. Determine cell number and viability by mixing 5 µL of cell suspension with 5 µL of trypan blue and using a hemocytomoter. Typically, $1 \times 10^6$ to $1.5 \times 10^6$ cells/mL can be harvested from one 25 cm² flask at 80–90% confluency.

**Note:** Do not use cells if the number of dead cells is greater than 5%.

iii. Centrifuge cells at $200 \times g$ for 3 minutes in a centrifuge with a swing-bucket rotor.

### 7. *Prepare Cells for Assay*

- *Time duration*: 20 minutes

Aspirate supernatant and resuspend cell pellet in a basal medium EBM-2 at a concentration of $1.5 \times 10^5$ cells/mL per 1 mL. The cells should be gently pipetted up and down a few times to obtain a single cell suspension.

## 8. *Prepare Cells for Addition of Test Materials*

- *Time duration*: 10–30 minutes
  i. Label four sterile 15 mL conical tube as follows: 35 nm mL 1 bFGF with 10 mM bFGF.
  ii. Load 1 mL ($1.5 \times 10^5$ cells) of a single cell suspension (step 6) in each tube. Centrifuge the tubes for 3 minutes at $200 \times g$ and aspirate the supernatent. Leftover cell suspension can either be discarded or seeded into 25 $cm^2$ cell culture flask in EGM-2 (complete growth medium) for future use.

**Note:** Do not disturb the cell pellets when aspirating supernatent. Invert the tube with single cell suspension a few times to prevent sedimentation of cells at the bottom of the tube.

  iii. Add the corresponding medium to cell pellets as follows: 3.5 µL of 10 ng µL$^{-1}$ with 10 mM bFGF and 1 mL complete medium EGM-2 and 1.5 µL of 10 mM sulforaphane stock solution.
  iv. Carefully resuspend cell pellets in the medium to make single cell suspensions at a concentration of $1.5 \times 10^5$ cells per mL.
  v. Carefully resuspend cell pellets in the medium to make single cell suspensions at a concentration of $1.5 \times 10^5$ cells per mL.

## 9. *Put Cells on Top of Gelled Basement Membrane Extract*

- *Time duration*: 15 minutes to add cells, 4–16 hours incubation time
  i. Gently add 100 µL (15,000 cells) per well of the single cell suspensions prepared in steps 7 and 8 to corresponding labeled wells of a 96-well plate on top of the gelled basement membrane extract.

**Note:** Be sure that cells are well mixed when adding them to the well, as cell density has an effect on tube formation. Do not touch the surface of the gel when adding the cells and add the cell suspension slowly so as not to injure the gelled material.

  ii. Incubate 96-well plate at 37°C, 5% $CO_2$ in the cell culture incubator for a period of 4–16 hours, or until the desired result is achieved. Examine the plate every hour for tube formation under an inverted microscope with ×4 or ×10 objective.

**Note:** During first hour of the tube assay, do not shake the plate or take it out of cell culture incubator. When observing the plate under a microscope, do not keep it longer than a minute or two outside the cell culture incubator.

## Observation

Once tube formation is observed, use the preferred option to obtain results. The following options can be employed depending on the equipment available:

i. *Microscopy*: Photograph the tubular network in the wells using a digital camera attached to an inverted microscope with X4 or X10 objective.

ii. *Macroscopy*: Aspirate the medium from the wells, add 100 µL of warm DPBS and immediately photograph the wells. Replacing the medium with DPBS solution can be necessary if the medium contains phenol red and the color reduces the quality of the pictures.

**Note:** Gently aspirate and load solutions so as not to disturb the network of endothelial cell tubes. Do not keep tubular network in DPBS for extended period of time, because it may detach from the matrix and start breaking apart.

iii. *Calcein AM*: Prepare 6 µM of calcein AM by adding 3 µL of 2 mM calcein AM stock solution to 1 mL EBM-2 medium. Without aspirating the medium, add 50 µL of 6 µM calcein AM solution per well of the 96-well plate. Incubate the plate at 37°C and in 5% $CO_2$ for 15–30 minutes. Calcein AM-labeled cells should be observed and photographed using a fluorescent inverted microscope with 485 nm excitation or 520 nm emission filter.

iv. *Fixation of endothelial cells to the basement membrane matrix followed by labeling with cell staining solution*: Aspirate the medium from the wells and rinse the wells 3 times with 100 µL of PBS per well. Aspirate the last wash, add 100 µL of –20°C cold methanol per well and incubate the plate for 30 seconds to 1 minute. Aspirate methanol and immediately rinse the wells 3 times with distilled $H_2O$. Aspirate last wash, add 100 µL of cell staining solution per well and incubate the plate for 15–30 minutes at room temperature (21°C). Rinse the wells 3 times with distilled $H_2O$. Endothelial cells can be photographed and images can be used for quantitation.

**Anticipitated results:** Examples of endothelial cells plated on top of the gelled reduced growth factor basement membrane extract (BME) with no stimulation of angiogenesis and with stimulated angiogenesis are shown in Fig. 8.12. In the absence of an angiogenic factor, just a few tubes are observed with disconnected networks (Fig. 8.12 A). In the presence of an angiogenic factor (10 mM bFGF), the cells attach, align and form tubes with a lumen that appears as a network (Fig. 8.12 B). Formation of tubular-like network is more profound in the presence of multiple angiogenic factors in the EGM-2 medium (Fig. 8.12 C). In the presence of an angiogenic factor

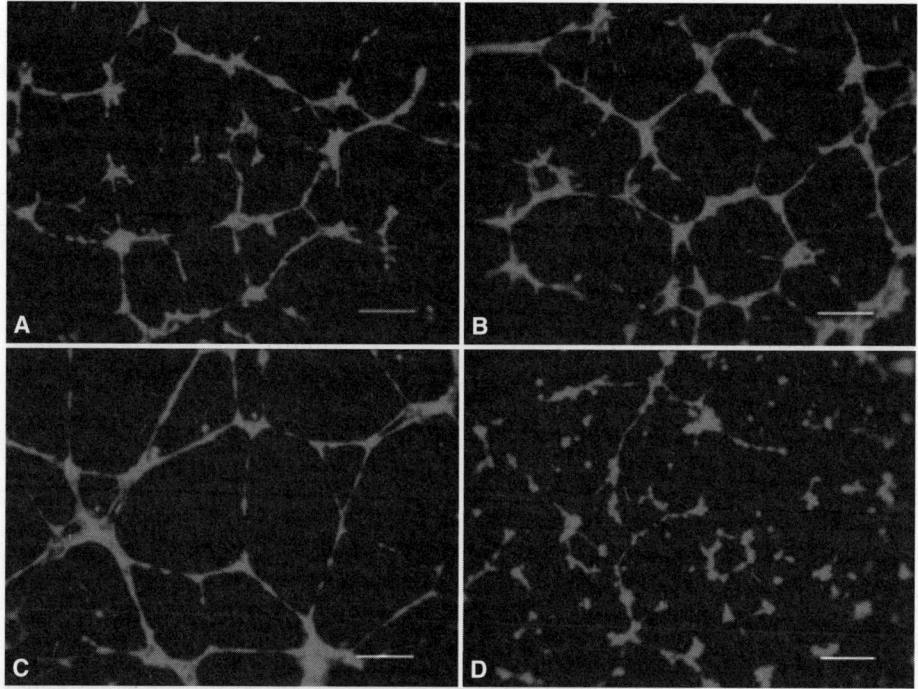

**Fig. 8.12A to D:** Effect of angiogenesis stimulators and an inhibitor on tube formation. Shown is the appearance of endothelial cell tubes on a basement membrane substratum in the (A) endothelial basal media-2 (EBM-2) without angiogenesis stimulators; (B) EBM-2 with 10 mM bFGF; (C) endothelial growth media (EGM-2) that contains 2% fetal bovine serum, hydrocortisone, bFGF, VEGF, R3-IGF, ascorbic acid, heparin, hEGF and GA-1000; and in the (D) EGM-2 with 15 µM of sulforaphane, an inhibitor of angiogenensis.

and an inhibitor of angiogenesis (15 µM sulforaphane), the cells attach and remain somewhat rounded as solitary cells (Fig. 8.12 D). The effect of the inhibitor is generally dose-dependent.

## Bibliography

1. Arnaoutova, I, and Kleinman, HK (2010). *In vitro* angiogenesis: endothelial cell tube formation on gelled basement membrane extract. Nature Protocols, 5(4), 628.
2. Foubert, P, Matrone, G, Souttou, B, Leré-Déan, C, Barateau, V, Plouët, J, and Tobelem, G (2008). Coadministration of endothelial and smooth muscle progenitor cells enhances the efficiency of proangiogenic cell-based therapy. Circulation Research, 103(7), 751–760.
3. Shen, JS, Meng, XL, Schiffmann, R, Brady, RO, and Kaneski, CR (2007). Establishment and characterization of Fabry disease endothelial cells with an extended lifespan. Molecular Genetics and Metabolism, 92(1), 137–144.

# Index

α-amylase inhibitory action 63
α-glucosidase inhibitory assay 65
β-lactamase inhibition assay 110
5-Lipoxygenase inhibition assay 23
72-h *in vitro* growth inhibition assay 131

**A**gar dilution method 106
Albumax 116, 131, 133
*Allium cepa* root tip assay 143
American Psychological Association style
   (APA) 11
Amies medium 84, 87
Angiogenesis 140, 173
Angiopoietins and tie receptors 174
Annexin A5 159, 163
Apoptosis 148

**B**asal media 84
Bioassay 1
Blood agar media 84, 85
Bordet-Gengou medium 87
Bracketing method 4
Broth dilution method 103, 108

**C**ampylobacter medium 87
Cancer 140
Cancer cell lines 141, 142
Cary-Blair medium 87
Charcoal-yeast agar 86
Chemotherapy 82
Chorioallantoic membrane assay (CAM) 177
Christensen's urea medium 87
Culture media 83, 88–90
Cyclo-oxygenase (COX) 28, 32
Cytotoxic potential 151, 153

**D**efined media 87
Deoxycholate citrate agar (DCA) 86
Diabetes mellitus (DM) 60
Differential medium 86, 89
Direct colony suspension method 96
Disc diffusion test 96
DNA fragmentation 154, 166

DPPH scavenging activity 42
Dubos medium 86

**E**nd point assay 4
Endothelial cell tube formation assay 180
Enriched media 84
Enrichment medium 89
Eosin-methylene blue (EMB) agar 86
Erythrocyte suspension 19, 117

**F**erric reducing antioxidant power (FRAP)
   assay 52
Fibroblast growth factor 175, 180

**G**ermination assay 146
Glucose diffusion assay 67
Glycation inhibition assay 71
Graded response assay 3

**H**arvard style of referencing 11
HbA1c 61
Heat-induced hemolysis 19
Hiss serum water medium 85
Human red blood cells (HRBC)
   suspension 19
Hyaluronidase inhibition assay 25
Hydrogen peroxide scavenging ($H_2O_2$)
   assay 44
Hydroxyl (HO·) radical scavenging 56
Hypotonicity-induced hemolysis 21

**I**ndicator (differential) media 84
Inflammation 14
Interpolation assay 4, 5

**K**irby-Bauer method 94
Kligler iron agar (KIA) 87

**L**eishmaniasis 112
Leshmaniacidal assay 138
Loeffler serum 86
Log dose response (LDR) curve 4
Log potency ratio 5
Log-rank test 8, 9

Lowenstein-Jensen medium  85
Luminescent assay protocol  29

**M**acConkey agar media  85
Malaria  113
Matching point method  4
McFarland standard  100
Membrane stabilization assay  19
Minimum bactericidal concentration
    (MBC)  108
Minimum inhibitory concentration
    (MIC)  106
Mitotic index  143, 144, 147
MLA citation style  12
Motility indole urea (MIU) medium  87
MTS cytotoxicity assays  150
MTT cytotoxicity assays  152
Müeller-Hinton agar media  85
Müeller-Hinton agar  94
Multi-point bioassay  5

**N**eovascularization  174
NICE  61
Nitric oxide scavenging activity  46
Nonparametric analysis  8
Nutridoma-SR  116
Nutrient agar media  84
Nutrient broth media  84

**O**ral glucose tolerance test (OGTT)  61

**P**eptone water media  85
Peptone water sugar media  85
Peroxidase assay  35
Phosphomolybdenum method  50
Platelet-derived growth factor (PDGF)  175
Protease inhibition assay  75
Protein denaturation  17, 18
Protein tyrosine phosphatase inhibition
    assay  69

**Q**ualitative bioassay  2
Quantal assay  4
Quantitative bioassays  2

**R**educing power method  48

**S**almonella-Shigella (SS) agar  86
Science citation index  13
Scientific citation  10
Selective media  84, 86
Selenite F broth  86
Slide staining  156
Starch iodine method  63
Statistical interference  7
Sterilization of culture media  92
Stokes method  100
Storage media  84
Superoxide radical scavenging assay  58

**T**ellurite blood agar  86
Tellurite-gelatin agar medium (TGAM)  87
Tetrathionate broth  86
The Chicago manual of style  12
The Kaplan-Meier method  8
Thiosulphate-citrate-bile-sucrose (TCBS)
    agar  86
Three-point assay  4
Transforming growth factors  174
Transport media  84
Tropical diseases  112
Tumor necrosis factor-$\alpha$  174
TUNEL assay  166
Tyrosinase inhibition assay  78

**V**ancouver style  12
Vascular endothelial growth factor  174

**X**anthine oxidase activity  54
Xylose lysine deoxycholate (XLD)  86